A Face To Meet The

Faces

Selected posts from the *Illusions of Autonomy* blog

By Philip Berry MD FRCP

Unless otherwise attributed, odd stick man illustrations are by the author.

Underlined 'hyperlinks' have been left in place from the blog; they link to free resources if an article is accessed on the blog website.

By the same author (available via Amazon as e-books or paperbacks)

Motives, emotion and memory - exploring how doctors think (1st blog collection)

Spoken/Unspoken - hidden mechanics of the patient-doctor relationship (2nd blog collection)

Proximity (Nina Charan medical thriller)

Extremis (2nd Nina Charan medical thriller)

The Pioneer

Malady/Therapy (short stories)

TABLE OF CONTENTS

INTRODUCTION 5

HOLLOW HEROES..8

SWITCHING OFF 12

A RARE AND UNPLEASANT DUTY: INVOLUNTARY TREATMENT AND THE
DEPRIVATION OF LIBERTY 17

INTERACTIVE WARD ETHICS 1: COLLUSION....................................26

THE PATIENT AS RIDDLE 61

SINGULAR HISTORIES, COMMON NEEDS: 71

REPLACING THE LCP 71

MAKING DEALS: THE PROBLEM OF THE SELF 80

DISCHARGING PATIENT 80

TEMPTING FATE: THE PERILS OF REASSURANCE 86

STUDENTS, YOU MAKE US BETTER DOCTORS 89

THE GOOD IN HIM..93

FRIGIDARIUM: ON POST-MORTEMS, AND TAKING THE PLUNGE....................101

MESSENGERS 104

A LITTLE PIECE OF YOU – CARE.DATA DIALOGUE 107

TWO ROOMS 118

INTERACTIVE WARD ETHICS 2: DANGEROUS 121

CANDOUR CRUNCH: BEING HONEST ABOUT RISKS ON HEALTHCARE.............154

NOTES ON A JUDGMENT 159

THE TURNING AWAY 171

PATTERNS AND PRIDE: DIARY OF MEDICAL ANECDOTE 174

A GIFT FREELY GIVEN: DIALOGUE ON ORGAN DONATION 182

LEADERSHIP – THE IMMEDIACY OF EXAMPLE 194

RIGHT TO BE WRONG: BEING COMFORTABLE WITH UNCERTAINTY 198

PATIENT COMPLAINTS AND THE RESPONSE ARC 203

HURRICANE KATRINA AND THE DNR FALLACY 209

BED X 215

INTERACTIVE WARD ETHICS 3: OBEDIENT 219

4

Introduction

This is the third collection of blog posts to be published since I started writing regularly in August 2012. The title of this book, *A Face to Meet The Faces,* represents a change of focus. I am interested in describing the workings of the medical mind - all the ticks, clicks, springs and processes that are engaged before the first word is spoken to a patient. I do not suggest that the face we present is insincere, but it is professional, and it will not express our every thought. Occasionally, as Dev finds in *'The good in him'*, those processes result in an entirely wrong impression being given to those whom a busy doctor is trying to help. At other times our usual natures and inhibitions are challenged by special situations, and we find ourselves *'Making deals'* (with patients who wish to self-discharge), or dancing along the fine line between treatment and bodily assault (*'A rare and unpleasant duty: involuntary treatment and the deprivation of liberty'*). Those normal natures can render us susceptible to pride (*'Diary of a medical anecdote'*, *'Hollow Heroes'*), expediency (*'The perils of reassurance'*) or paralyzing timidity (*'Being comfortable with uncertainty'*).

Elsewhere, subjects have grabbed my attention randomly (the Hurricane Katrina healthcare catastrophe for instance), or I have reacted to observations in the media (*'Bed X'*), or to important policy developments (such as changes in organ donation). The core preoccupations that fuelled the first two collections - end of life care, autonomy, resuscitation decisions, the Liverpool Care Pathway, medical futility – are still represented (*Replacing the LCP, Notes on a judgment*).

A new feature is the 'ethical adventure' or *Interactive Ward Ethics* section - a role playing, decision making exercise inspired by the Fighting Fantasy books I read as a child. The reader is asked to decide, on behalf of the well-meaning and conscientious young doctor Nina, what to do in a variety of challenging situations. There are three in this volume, and the idea is to roam vicariously through the actions of a sometimes luckless substitute!

It can do no harm to illustrate how we sometimes struggle to accommodate the emotional dissonances encountered in healthcare, although I do not pretend to set out solutions. The first, most important step, it seems to me, is identifying the challenges. I hope this collection of articles serves that purpose.

There will be time, there will be time

To prepare a face to meet the faces that you meet

(From The Love-Song of J. Alfred Prufrock, by T.S. Eliot)

oOo

I am, as ever, hugely grateful to readers who follow my blog, and to my followers on Twitter who spread the word about particular posts when my writing hits the mark. Thanks also to my lovely wife Kirsty, and to my children who go to bed on time thus leaving the evenings free for all of this!

Hollow heroes

Justifiably or not, young doctors are inspired and motivated by the thought that they might, one day, save somebody's life. Opportunities come rarely, but spend long enough in a hospital and one day you will find yourself in a situation where a single action (be it a procedure, a prescription or a revelatory, previously un-thought of diagnosis) will stop a patient from dying in front of you. You cannot help but walk away immensely pleased, brimming with adrenaline enhanced satisfaction.

Some would say the temptation to wallow in a bath of warm aggrandisement is self-centred. It may encourage a too narrow perception of the clinical encounter, diminishing the suffering or fear felt by the patient and magnifying the importance of the doctor. For after all, who really matters here, you or the person who's life has been saved? But I would defend the doctor who excitedly recounts such an episode to a friends or partner by inserting *themselves* in the lead role, because to suppress that pleasure, and take the puritanical view that 'it's just my job, it means nothing' would be to deny doctors access to a very important source of job satisfaction. However, experience has told me that there is a quid pro quo, one that is revealed when things go badly. We must ask ourselves – how happy are we to take the lead role when our actions or omissions contributed to suffering…or even death?

My SHO and I (a registrar at the time) were called to see a patient with cirrhosis who had started to vomit blood. We resuscitated him, decided it was safe to take him down for an endoscopy, and within half an hour we were watching the varix spurting blood across the field of view on the monitor. I fired two bands, the bleeding stopped, and the drama was over. My SHO looked across, still squeezing the second bag of blood and clearly impressed, and said,

"You just saved his life." What impressed him, I think, was not my specific role in this, but the fact that a procedure could so swiftly stabilise a patient. The experience would prove a clincher for him…he had been thinking about choosing this specialty and the opportunity to perform heroics, like this, was just what he needed to witness.

But as we walked back to the ward I began to explain,

"It's not me, or us, who saved him. If *we* weren't here today there would be another registrar, and another SHO, who would have found him and 'scoped him. The chances are they would have done just as good a job."

"But it was you. You made the diagnosis and sorted everything out."

"But those were not exceptional actions. They are just what you do in those circumstances."

"You may as well give yourself a bit of a pat on the back."

"I am, internally, because I'm glad we made all the right decisions. But what we did was *normal*. We are working in a system that is designed to allow us to find patients who need us to apply our training and skills, so really it's the system that saved the patient. Not us personally."

"So you don't get any fundamental satisfaction from that?"

"I do, but I have to put it into perspective. So do you. Try this. Imagine we had got the patient down here…no…imagine YOU were the registrar and had got the patient down here. And imagine you were doing the endoscopy, found the varix, but messed up somehow. You didn't set up the banding kit properly, or you chose the wrong place to band. And he kept bleeding. Then he vomited blood and aspirated, then had a respiratory arrest and died in front of you. How would you feel?"

"Awful."

"And would you blame yourself?"

"Yes."

"Really?"

"Of course I would, if I messed up."

"Up to a point. But I think I know what your mind would do. Everybody does the same. You feel bad, you go home, you think on it, you talk to your mates…then you rationalise. -- He was in a high risk group -- The endoscopy nurse should have told me the banding kit was not set up correctly -- In fact she should have set it up anyway -- There wasn't time to arrange anaesthetic support -- The varices must have been under high pressure -- These patients, what do they expect when they drink all their lives? --…"

"I would never think that."

"The mind can go to some dark places when you feel under threat."

"I wouldn't just rationalise it away."

"Perhaps, to some extent, just to keep yourself functional. My point is, whenever you are tempted to congratulate yourself on a job well done, imagine how prominently placed you would want to see yourself in the scene if things hadn't gone well."

"It sounds very joyless."

"A bit. My advice is, enjoy the satisfaction, but don't talk about it. Because fate has a way of arranging things so that after every example of brilliance or skill, something comes along to bring you straight back down to earth."

Switching off

It was the day before Christmas. Matt was a FY2* working in an acute Trust. His registrar explained,

'Our job, today, is to set a course for each of our patients, make sure their treatment is right, resuscitation and escalation decisions considered, frequency of reviews agreed and handed over...'

'We're only away for a couple of days.'

'I know. Easter is worse actually. But the hospital won't be running at full tilt between Christmas and New Year, and I'm taking one day off, Suzy's seeing her family in the States - she was lucky to get that agreed but her Mum's ill I think - and for good or bad, it's the sickest ones that will get most of the attention. So go to it! I'm in clinic, but I'll check in afterwards.'

Matt and the FY1 saw everyone and made clear plans, but late in the day he picked up a few complications and serious developments. He left at 7.45PM and found the roads deserted. Most workers were home already, but he had a three hour drive ahead of him. As he drove he thought about two patients for whom he had prescribed new treatment, one with pneumonia, the other with renal failure and dangerously high potassium levels. It was still quite a novel experience for him to make a firm diagnosis and start treatment without direct supervision, but by quarter to eight on Christmas Eve the wards were not exactly overrun with seniors. To be fair, at 6.30PM all had seemed settled, and he had said goodbye to his registrar with confidence and goodwill!

When he woke up on Christmas morning, in his parent's house, the first things to enter his mind were the two patients he had treated just twelve hours before. Both should have been reviewed at around midnight, the one with renal failure requiring a repeat potassium check, the one with pneumonia a blood gas. Matt had handed both tasks over, but he was concerned. When he made the hand over call, the evening SHO was being gradually buried in last minute requests as each team tried to leave for the holidays. Matt went downstairs and joined his two siblings, one older and one younger, and his parents for breakfast. This would be the last year that they spent Christmas together - there were babies and partners and houses and grown up commitments coming. He enjoyed the meal, but the thought of the renal failure patient kept nagging at him. He must have appeared distracted, for his father commented,

'What's on your mind son?'

'Oh, nothing...work.'

'Well, you're off now aren't you. The poor sods who are in today can deal with it.'

'Yes...but...' and he didn't go into it. His father was not in healthcare, he had been a successful businessman who's company seemed to shut down entirely for two weeks over Christmas. Matt remembered that he had brought work home for the holidays, and, thinking about it, there must have been worries and concerns that niggled even though the doors were closed. But his father had always hid them well, committing himself fully to the time the family spent together. Perhaps Matt had to learn the skill – that of closing out his professional life for a couple of days and appearing relaxed. Perhaps he would learn not only to appear relaxed, but to *be* relaxed!

They had lunch, and the two glasses of Prosecco spurred him into a mood a conviviality, but as he sat down on the sofa at 3PM and let his eyelids fall, a fluorescent green line flashed into his mind's eye and scurried across the dark field. His renal patient, in cardiac arrest! It was now time for presents. Again, he must have put on a poor show, because his sister took him to one side and asked,

'What is it? You look miles away.'

Matt told her. She was unimpressed,

'It's not your concern. You're off now. Come on...'

'I've got to know what has happened to him.'

'You'll find out when you go back won't you?'

'I suppose so.'

He went back into the lounge, but fifteen minutes later said he was going to the loo and went upstairs. Covertly, in a whisper, he used his mobile phone to ring the hospital switchboard. He waited eight minutes and 47 seconds (his mobile display ticked over silently and patiently) to get through. He guessed that many relatives were trying to contact wards to check that their interned loved ones were alright. After another five minutes the on-call house officer answered her bleep. Matt asked her if she had seen his renal patient. She hadn't.

'Hang on...' she said, 'I'll check the computer for something, the name rings a bell.' A pause, keyboard taps. 'He's on intensive care. Oh yes! I remember, I heard all about it when I arrived this morning. He was reviewed at 2AM and his potassium was over seven or eight something...the house officer on overnight called ITU, they came to see him, and an hour later he was on a filter. He's fine. Good job he was reviewed. Could have done with being seen a bit sooner probably...his ECG was horrible, they think he was two hours away from arresting, he was so acidotic too. Was he your patient?'

'Yes...I arranged the review...'

'Good thing you did...'

'Thanks. Thanks for answering.'

'Why are you ringing, it's Christmas day?'

'I just…wanted to know...'

'Relax man! We've got it covered. Go and get drunk.'

And he did. Later he dreamt of ships arriving in harbour, their cargo safe, all hands present.

– – –

* FY2 = doctor who has been qualified for 1 year

A rare and unpleasant duty: involuntary treatment and the deprivation of liberty

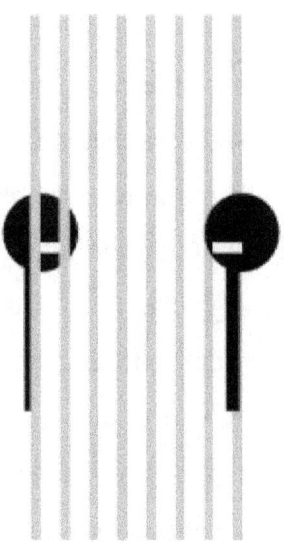

One of the most disturbing and unexpected duties of a doctor in training is that of depriving a person of their liberty.

The following scenario describes the emotional and intellectual challenges involved in sedating someone against their will to keep them in hospital. It is worth remembering that the doctors asked to deal with these situations can be junior and inexperienced. Their exposure to the legal frameworks that permit a doctor to do legally what only judges, police officers, prison warders, soldiers and psychiatrists do routinely, may amount to no more than 15 minutes during induction or the fading memories of a lecture three years before they qualified.

A 75 year old man with early dementia (which has had little effect on his life or degree of independence thus far) is admitted to hospital. He may have a mild chest infection, and is on intravenous antibiotics, but it's one of those diagnoses that is made more because something "must be going on" than due to solid clinical evidence. During the night following his admission the house officer on call is asked to attend the ward urgently. The man is trying to self-discharge. The doctor, Paul, is used to this, although he is usually asked to dissuade younger patients, such as the alcohol addicted, those who regard themselves as indestructible or, sometimes, high-flyers who just 'don't have time' to be sick! He sits with the man, and hears how he is worried about his wife at home, unconvinced that he really needs to be here, unhappy with the whole 'overreaction'. He is a bit agitated, but asks, quite sensibly and insightfully, if his medications can't be delivered in tablet form. Paul thinks he has a point, but it's the middle of the night and it would be crazy to start arranging discharge. Any anyway, when he looks at the blood results there are some very high inflammatory markers; there may be more going on medically than meets the eye. Paul seems to succeed in reassuring the patient, he agrees to stay, and that's that.

The same ward calls Paul at 3AM. The patient is raging, marching up and down the ward in a highly agitated state; he has sworn and shouted, and he has cracked a pain of reinforced glass in the main door (which the nurse on charge locked during the build up). There are two security guards on the ward already, hanging back a few yards, not wishing to inflame the situation but ready to restrain him if necessary. Paul, a head shorter than the patient but over 50 years his junior, looks around him. Other patients are awake, some are equally as confused and relatively oblivious, some are young adults who are clearly horrified by the spectacle.

Paul talks to the patient, but the nursing staff have already tried reassurance and calm words without success. The patient pauses in his bubble of discomfort, indignity and despair, ringed by anxious faces and the muscle of the security guards. Paul asks him to go back to his bed space, but the words don't seem to be heard. Paul approaches and attempts to lay a hand on the patient's own hand, but immediately his arms rise and he begins to push away whatever spectres and threats he sees before him. The house officer perceives uncommon strength in the muscle of those arms, and knows from experience that delirium can lend the frailest patients the vigour of youth.

For this *must* be delirium. A usually calm man comes into hospital, wakes up in unfamiliar surroundings and tries to get home. His thoughts are clouded by the products of infection, cytokines, myriad substances, and, disinhibited, he does what he has never done in his life and breaks a window pane.

Then things deteriorate. The patient charges forward, collides with the resuscitation trolley, grabs it and swings it out into the corridor. Boxes fly onto the floor, a drip stand topples. He smacks another window but does not break it. He reacts to the pain. It is now getting out of hand. Paul knows what must be done. He instructs security to hold the patient and take him to his bed space. By this time there is a third member, and between them they pinion the patient and drag him away. The house officer looks around at the other patients, at their wide eyes in the dimmed light, and wonders how this looks. Once on the bed the patient begins to scream, for his every effort is met by opposition. A nurse has already gone for the lorazepam, and now presents the house officer with a two ml syringe containing 1mg of that drug diluted in one ml of saline.

Paul identifies the place where he will give the injection and asks the security guards to keep him as still as possible. Gently, Paul exposes an area of thigh, quickly wipes the skin and plunges the needle. He kneads the muscle for a few seconds, encouraging absorption, and hopes that it will begin to take effect soon. It does, miraculously. The tone leaves his patient's limbs and his vigour drains away. A nurse thanks Paul and the activity around the bed subsides. Good job.

But it was not so simple. While he was preparing the skin and preparing himself for the injection, Paul paused. He looked at the patient's face and listened to his words. The elderly man was articulating clearly, saying things like 'Don't let them do this' and 'Take me home' and '*Why* are you letting them do this?'

Taken in isolation each cry and phrase appeared to reveal a very clear intent, a transparent desire not to be here, not to be sedated and controlled. Every planned action in Paul's stressed mind was contrary to the patient's wishes. But he knew that he must give the injection because the patient really was not of sound mind at this time. He was delirious, he had no mental capacity. He was 'incapacitate' and a danger to himself, let alone others. As he brought the syringe close to the skin, Paul sensed a sudden relaxation, and looked up at the patient's face. His eyes, boring into those of the young doctor's, communicated a depth of emotion and desire that was hard to ignore. They were the same eyes, windows into the same mind, that two hours previously had explained in logical terms why he wanted to go home. Perhaps this was just anger. Haven't we all 'lost it', as children, after a punch on the nose or a terrible taunting. Wasn't he just extremely frustrated, able to see no other way out. Perhaps, having tried reason, he could no more than scream and fight. Was this truly a loss of capacity?

During the pause Paul asked himself if what he was doing was *right*. He quickly ran through the mental capacity checklist:

Can he understand what we're saying to him?

Can he retain that information long enough to be able to make a decision?

Can he weigh up that information and understand the consequences of his decision?

Can he communicate his decision?

Well, Paul thought, let's consider this. Understand - why not, who is to say. He could before. Retain? We're not really giving him the time to test that are we. Weigh up? That's pretty subjective...he already told me what he thought about the risks of going home versus staying in hospital, when we met earlier. It's the same decision he's being asked to consider now, and his point of view has evidently not changed. And communicate? Hell yes, he's communicating in every conceivable way. So is he really incapacitate? I can't absolutely, with complete and utter confidence, say that he does not. But as he bucks and shouts under the well-trained restraint provided by 'security', this intellectual debate seems irrelevant. If I don't do something he will stand up, charge out of the ward in his night clothes and run through the car park into the road. There is no question as to what is right. I *must* sedate him in his best interests.

As Paul walks away from the ward into the numerous tasks that must be completed before the sun rises, he comforts himself. Of course it was right. Any right thinking doctor would have done the same. But this challenge positioned him in absolute opposition to the expressed desires of his patient. This was worse than causing pain by messing up venflons; it was more distressing, in its immediacy and philosophical distastefulness, than telling someone they have cancer.

oOo

In the field of psychiatry, where involuntary detention and treatment is a common enough demand, there is a well established and well rehearsed legal framework to guide practitioners and protect patients (the Mental Health Act). In the field of general medicine, where physical illness can impair cognitive function, things are less clear, although efforts have been made over the last decade to draft appropriate laws and make their application straightforward. The Mental Capacity Act 2005, and its Deprivation Of Liberty Safeguards (DOLS) addition (2009) are realistic and practical. As described on the Alzheimer's Society website,

'In an emergency, the management of the hospital or care home may grant itself an urgent authorisation, but must apply for a standard authorisation at the same time. This urgent authorisation is usually valid for seven days, although the supervisory body may extend this for up to another seven days in some circumstances. Before an urgent authorisation is given, steps should be taken to consult with carers and family members.'

The DoLS legislation appears aimed more at ongoing situations where individuals are re-located against their will, locked in, their movements and activity controlled. In fact DoLS legislation was brought about in response to the 'Bournewood case' (well described in this European Human Rights Commission webpage) in which a man with autism was kept in hospital for treatment that doctors felt was in best interests. His usual carers complained and took the hospital to court. The government, seeing that there was a legal gap whereby reasonable deprivation of liberty could not be legal, enacted DoLS.

However, what we as doctors are often asked to do on-call or in the emergency department may not amount to deprivation of liberty. It may feel like it, but 'restraining or restricting' a patient in their best interests may not require DoLS to be invoked. There is a role for common sense applied urgently and safely. As described on the legal firm Morgan Cole's website,

Restraint or restrictions on an incapacitate individual's liberty can be justified under the Mental Capacity Act 2005 provided:

- reasonable steps are taken to establish that the individual lacks capacity in relation to the matter in question; and

- it is reasonably believed that the individual does lack capacity in relation to the matter in question; and

- it is in the best interests of that individual for the act to be done; and

- it is reasonably believed that it is necessary to do the act to prevent harm to that individual; and

- the act in question is a proportionate response to the likelihood of the individual suffering harm; and

- the act in question is a proportionate response to the seriousness of that harm

Paul and his patient seemed to meet these considerations, but the thinking and empathic doctor, highly trained in the art of understanding a patient's plight, listening to their words and seeing their point of view, will never find it easy.

Interactive Ward Ethics 1: Collusion

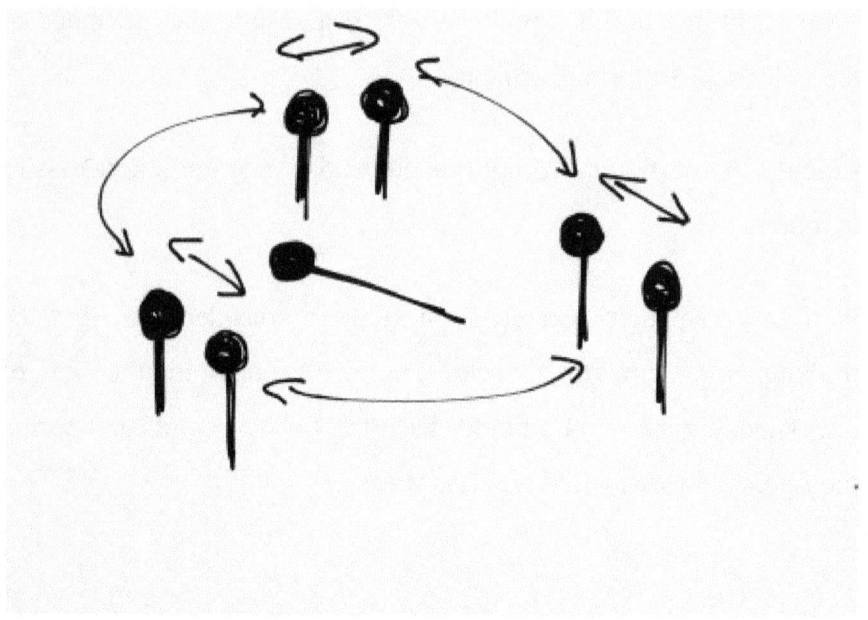

This is the first interactive medical ethics adventure to be published on the Illusions of Autonomy blog. You will guide an experienced trainee doctor, Nina Charan, through a difficult but not uncommon scenario, and in exploring the consequences of various decisions will experience the risks and pitfalls that are encountered on medical wards. It may end after just two decisions, or it may require 5 or 6 to reach a conclusion. Feel free to flip back and forth. It's not really about getting to the end - more the ups and downs that occur on the way.

The first scenario concerns an elderly lady whose son forbids the medical team to tell her about a serious diagnosis.

Good luck!

oOo

1.

Nina read the notes and prepared to see the patient. An 82 year old lady, Dorothy Lewis, was admitted overnight with abdominal swelling, but with no significant past medical problems. An ultrasound scan had already been requested and performed, the previous evening – it showed multiple liver lesions, likely metastatic cancer deposits. There appeared to be no history of dementia, and already Nina could see that patient was sitting out and reading a newspaper. She paused, considered what words to use, and walked to the bed space.

Just as she arrived at the end of the patient's bed a nurse touched her shoulder and beckoned her back to the nurses' station,

"Nina, her son just called, he was in a bit of a state. He said that no-one should talk to his Mum about the results of any tests until he has arrived."

Speak to the patient and tell her the result - go to 2

Speak to the patient, tell her the result only if she asks for it – go to 3

Speak to the patient, but withhold the result – go to 4

2.

After some general questions, and an examination (the liver could be felt, knobbly and hard) Nina mentioned the USS scan. The nurse was standing to one side, while Nina perched on the bed.

"Yes, I had it last night." said Dorothy.

"There were some abnormalities on it."

"Really, what?"

"They look suspicious, they may be tumours…a type of cancer, possibly. In fact I think that is the most likely explanation, that it has spread from somewhere else in the body…" Nina felt that she had spoken poorly, unsettled by the message from the son – nerves. Dorothy stared across the bed space, frozen. Nina touched her hand, seeming to awake her.

Dorothy said,

"My son. Where's my son? WHERE'S MY SON?"

The nurse shook her head, and just as Nina stood up to go the curtain parted and Dorothy's son appeared, incensed.

"What have you told her?" Dorothy answered for Nina,

"They think I've got cancer…just like that…just like your father…"

The son shook his head, sat next to his mother, and embraced her shoulders. He glanced up at Nina, and she perceived a sense of betrayal in his eyes.

Go to 5

3.

After some general questions, and an examination (the liver could be felt, knobbly and hard), Nina began to talk about what should be done next, the kind of investigations that would be needed. She did not mention the scan.

"What about the scan I had last night?" asked Dorothy. Nina hesitated,

"Would you like someone here with you, when we discuss your results with you? Sometimes it helps."

"My son would like to be here, if it's complicated. But he works. He'll be at work now, up in town."

"OK. Well, we can wait for him to come, or call him in. There are some things you, and he, need to know."

"I'll leave it to you to decide doctor. It sounds important."

"OK. We've seen the result of you scan, and were some abnormalities on it."

"Really, what abnormalities?"

"They look suspicious, for cancer possibly. In fact I think that is the most likely explanation, that it has spread from somewhere else in the body…"

Dorothy stared across the bed space, frozen. Nina touched her hand, seeming to awake her. Dorothy said,

"Oh God. Not like my Stan, please not like him…" Then she began to cry. The nurse shook her head, and just as Nina stood up to go the curtain parted and Dorothy's son appeared, incensed.

"What have you told her?"

"They think I've got cancer…like your father had…"

The son shook his head, sat next to his mother, and embraced her shoulders. He glanced up at Nina, and she saw a sense of betrayal in his eyes.

Go to 5

4.

After some general questions, and an examination (the liver could be felt, knobbly and hard) Nina paused. She had figured out what to say. The nurse was standing to one side, while Nina perched on the bed. Dorothy asked,

"It's swollen isn't it?"

"Yes, it is enlarged."

"So what did the scan I had last night show?"

"Well…" Nina paused, and made a decision…to lie, "the final result of it hasn't been given to us yet, sometimes the doctor who does the scan needs to review the pictures you see…we should have it back later."

"That's strange, he said the report would go onto the computers right away, he was going to speak into some sort of typing machine. He looked worried."

"We'll go and chase it…it won't be long. Is there anyone you would like here with you when we come to discuss results?"

"My son I'm sure would like to be here, but he works, and I'm quite capable of understanding anything you have to tell me."

Go to 6

5.

Dorothy's son stood in the ward. Nina recognised that this discussion could not be had here, and beckoned him into a private room. He spoke first,

"What you don't know, because you didn't think to wait to find out, was that my mother went through a terrible time when her husband, my father, was diagnosed. He was left alone for days, she was away herself, this was 30 years ago, no mobiles, no email. And when she came back he was desperate, and she never forgave herself....You should not have told her; she will slip back into severe depression...it will take away her will to live. I told you...I TOLD YOU!"

"We can't hide it from her forever, she needs to understand why we are making decisions, doing biopsies and things like that."

"Forever! What is that? Why do you need biopsies?"

"I think we do, to prove the diagnosis, and see if there is any treatment that might work help."

"Chemo you mean."

"Probably."

"She wouldn't want it. My father had that."

"But we need to hear her own thoughts on that."

"She's 82! What good will it do?"

"Some treatments are quite gentle nowadays."

"What does it involve?"

"Some local anaesthetic in the skin, and a very narrow needle into the liver for just a second."

"You need to do this?"

"To prove the diagnosis yes. Our oncologist will see her, but if he feels treatment would help…and I think he might, because she is otherwise very strong…then a biopsy will be recommended."

"*If* it shows cancer, *then* we can discuss what to tell her – if anything. But she is NOT to be told that she has a terminal illness, and anything you want to tell her *must* go through me first."

Agree to this condition and proceed with oncology referral, go to 7

Challenge the son, go to 19

6.

Nina sighed. She had lied. This was a first for her. She saw a few more patients, but half-heartedly. Then Dorothy's son arrived on the ward, and the two of them went to a private room. Her son, Brian, quickly established that his mother had been protected from the news of her scan result. Nina challenged him,

"Mr Lewis, I can't see this situation carrying on. She has her mental faculties, she will need to understand why we are doing more tests, perhaps internal camera tests, endoscopies, and keeping her in. It's not a sustainable situation, all the nurses and all the doctors will know what the true diagnosis is, but she won't. She may find out, accidentally. That will cause her more distress than if we sit with her, and talk to her."

"No. You don't know what it will do to her. I know her best, not you."

"It's hard for you too, I understand that. Let's leave things for now, and talk again in a day or two."

"That's fine. But as it stands, SHE IS NOT TO BE TOLD."

Go to 8

7.

Nina met the oncologist in the corridor at lunchtime. He headed up the Acute Oncology Service, and would review Dorothy the next day. But Nina wanted to get his rough opinion, and she described her patient. He pressed her on Dorothy's performance status, i.e. her physical strength, her independence on the ward, her social support. The impression was, pretty good…for now. Good enough for him to consider palliative chemotherapy. But there was a catch.

"I need to see histology before I plan treatment. Can you get a liver biopsy arranged today or tomorrow?"

"I'm sure we can."

Got to 13

8.

Nina happened to be on call the following night. She was called to her own ward at 3AM. Dorothy was triggering on the early warning score. Nina assessed her, and concluded that she had developed pneumonia. Antibiotics were prescribed, an oxygen mask attached, and things began to look a little better. Nina looked up the number of Dorothy's son, and sat with her finger on the dial buttons, in two minds. Would he want to know? – yes. Would he accept his mother's deterioration and agree to the limits of care that now seemed appropriate? – very likely. And the resuscitation status…that too. But then Nina looked across the ward, and saw how Dorothy was seeming to pick up and become more alert. She was lucid, she had mental capacity. She had to be involved in the resuscitation discussion. To exclude her from it seemed a step too far, a far more grave deception than withholding the cancer diagnosis.

She hesitated, not wanting to fall further into this game of collusion. Wait until the morning. But Nina would go home then, nothing would have been achieved. So she rang. There was no answer. She rang the mobile. A message. 'I am out of the country at the moment, I will get back to you as soon as possible.'

Dawn broke silently, and Nina noticed that the exterior windows, mirrors to her incessant overnight labours, now had an orange tinge. She came back to the ward at 8.30AM and discussed with her team whether the time had come to tell Dorothy everything. She was clearly dying, and unfit for anything but palliative care.

Tell the patient what her diagnosis is, discuss DNAR and refer to palliative care, go to 9

Commence palliative care measures but withhold diagnosis, go to 10

9.

"Mrs Lewis. Are you awake?"

She opened her eyes with difficulty, for the lids were sticky and dry from the oxygen rich air that escaped from the sides of the mask. She nodded. Nina tried to put herself well within Dorothy's field of view.

"You were very ill overnight. Do you remember me visiting you."

"Some of it. You jabbed me with a needle."

"I did, I'm sorry. You've got a chest infection."

"You can treat it."

"We are treating it, but you are very weak at the moment. It will be difficult for your "

"I'm sure it will. I'm old now."

"But more than that. I think we need…I need…to tell you more about what we've found out since you came in. The scan you had, it showed that there's a serious problem, in your liver. I think you might have cancer."

"Oh no."

"I know…your son said…that your husband had it too. But I can't hide it from you. This lung infection has happened because your defences are low. It might get worse. We need to talk about what to do, how to treat you."

"I need to have my son here."

"I'm not sure when he's coming in."

"I'm tired."

"I'll leave you. I'm going to ask some other doctors and nurses to see you this morning. They are very good at helping patients with cancer, when it looks like it cannot be cured…" But Dorothy seemed to have dropped off. Perhaps she had just turned off.

Refer to palliative care, go to 11

10.

Nina had recognised that Dorothy was dying. The antibiotics might forestall things for a short while, but there was a tinge of jaundice, and the liver tests showed that its infiltration was worsening rapidly. The right thing to do was concentrate on comfort. So she spoke to the nurse looking after her, asked that emergency calls not be out if her physiological parameters deteriorated, and confirmed that she was *Not For Cardiopulmonary Resuscitation*. When Nina sat down to complete the DNR form, she hesitated, troubled by the thought that Dorothy did have capacity to be involved in the discussion but was being excluded. Nina wrote something on the form to explain the particulars of the situation, and reassured herself that there was no question, absolutely no question, that the DNR decision was correct. This done, she picked up the phone to call palliative care.

Go to 12

11.

At 1PM the palliative care team arrived on the ward, comprising the specialist nurse and a consultant. They reviewed the notes and introduced themselves to the patient. They asked Dorothy what she wanted. By now she was asleep and uncommunicative for most of the hours of the day, but she was able to focus briefly on the conversation. The answer was – take me home. Her son appeared overcome with the pace of events, but did not refuse or complain. The force of nature appeared to have robbed him of the intensity that had shocked the ward staff. She went home 48 hours later, and Nina heard nothing more about her, or her son.

Go to Summing Up

12.

"She's probably in the last week of her life. Could you come to review her, perhaps talk about a supported discharge. She's widowed, but there's a son who lives to far away."

"And she knows the diagnosis?"

"Well, we haven't done a biopsy to get histology, but the scans are clear."

"So she knows she's got terminal cancer?"

"…errr…well, there's been a problem on that front. Her son has forbidden us to tell her."

"You've challenged that?"

"Up to a point, but he's absolutely convinced it will cause her distress."

"Of course it will…but we can't come and talk to her about dying of cancer unless you have told her first. You need to have more discussions with her son and try to explain why it's important to tell her, for her sake."

"And if we don't, she won't get any palliative care?"

"She will get the right care I'm sure, but she won't know why things are happening, and she'll die in ignorance. That may be right for her, I don't know, but I'm afraid the palliative care team is unlikely to be involved. How can we visit, how can we explain who we are?"

"Oh."

Manage patient alone, continue to withhold diagnosis, Go to 20

Find son, explore his concerns further and argue in favour of full disclosure, go to 23

13.

So Nina made the arrangements, and that afternoon Dorothy was wheeled down to the radiology department. Ten minutes later Nina's bleep went off, and she was summoned to the same department. A senior radiologist was standing, waiting for her, outside an ultrasound room. He was clearly upset.

"Dr Charan. You nearly had a hell of a situation on your hands here! Your patient, Dorothy Lewis. I was consenting her for a liver biopsy, and was explaining the purpose, which was to determine what sort of tumour she has in her liver so you guys can plan some treatment. It took her completely by surprise. She has no intention of having chemo…so there is no point doing something as invasive as this. In fact, listening to her, she seems to have made up her mind to die. She's completely compos mentis! Anyway, I've got a huge list, and I'm going to ask you to clear up this mess. If you want a biopsy you need to tell her what it's for."

Try to convince the radiologist to go ahead anyway, go to 14

Return to base, go to 15

14.

"Dr Stanton, we've made a considered decision here. I should have come down to forewarn you, but biopsy is felt to be essential, so that we can explore all the options. Her son thinks she'll crumble if we are explicit about all the details, the treatments and prognosis. He thinks she won't manage at all, and that any time she does have left will be blighted by depression and some sort of guilt she feels over her husband's death."

"And this has been agreed, with him, her next of kin?"

"Yes."

"OK, I'll do it. But if you don't do anything with the information it gives, then you've put her through something she didn't need, and the risk…small as it is. Not to mention our time!"

"Thank you Dr Stanton. It's so complicated."

Go to 16

15.

Nina wandered back to the ward. No biopsy, no further on. Perhaps chemotherapy was always unrealistic. Perhaps the best thing was for her to go home. But how, and with what support? Just her and her son, the two of them evading the truth until she began to deteriorate. Then the GP would be called in, and would be horrified to find the situation had been left unresolved. Dorothy needed the help of the palliative care team. That was what to do next.

Go to 24

16.

Two hours after returning to the ward Dorothy's blood pressure dropped. She developed some pain in the shoulder. Nina reviewed her, and recognised the signs of bleeding. She could not believe that this complication, so unusual nowadays, could happen to this patient.

"What's happening?" asked Dorothy.

"I think you are bleeding from the liver. From the biopsy."

"Oh dear. What can you do? It hurts."

"We can usually stop it, it involves going back to the department where you had it, so they can find the artery in the liver and block it."

Nina rang Dr Stanton, the radiologist.

"I looked at the liver again Nina, when I did the biopsy. It's full of tumour, full of it. It must be very vascular. They aren't so easy to embolise. Perhaps you should leave her alone now."

"I don't think we're at that stage Dr Stanton."

"Well if she comes back down here she needs to know why and what's happening to her. If it gets complicated she will hear the word cancer, she'll see everyone running around, we won't be able to pussy foot around it. Tell her what she needs to know. Tell her, or I'm not taking her back, it's not fair on any of us, let alone the patient."

Tell her, go to 17

Withhold, and contact her son, go to 18

17.

"Mrs Lewis, we've got to get you downstairs right away."

"Good, good. I don't feel well at all."

"But I must tell you what's happening…I wish your son were here, but this is quite an emergency now, and it's really necessary for you to know what is happening to you. We can't not tell you."

"I understand Dr Charan. I do. So tell me. It's terminal, isn't it?"

"It is, we think."

"I knew. Of course I knew. I saw it in all your eyes."

"Are you angry at us, for not telling you."

"No, of course not. Because I knew. And because I trust my son. I don't want to linger on. I don't want anything more. Ask my son to come in, please."

Nina walked away. Her patient was bleeding to death, an iatrogenic condition, a complication, of a procedure she didn't even want or need. Nina would have difficulty explaining this. She had messed it up. Messed it up right at the beginning and made the wrong decision.

Go to Summing Up

18.

Nina called the contact number in Dorothy's notes. Her son answered promptly, and Nina explained the situation. It had become imperative, in the medical team's opinion, to share details of the diagnosis with the patient.

"Wait, don't do anything, I'm coming in."

"How long will you be."

"An hour and a half, door to door."

"That's too long."

"Don't tell her. I have to be there."

"I need to tell her now, or the bleeding will continue…"

"So take her."

"It's not simple, it's a complicated procedure, and if it doesn't work, she could…"

"What? Die?"

"Yes. And she would die without knowing why."

"She would prefer it that way."

Nina had no answer. She did not have the confidence or the experience, in this situation, to invoke the law. She prevaricated.

"I will need to take her down in 90 minutes from now. If you are not here by then, I will take her."

"So be it. I'll be there."

Go to 22

19.

"What happened to her, with the depression?"

"She spent 6 months in an…institution. This was in the 1980's. She had electroconvulsive therapy, to bring her out of a catatonic state. They delved into her mind, traced it back to my father's diagnosis. After she came home – I was at university during this period – she was not the same. Whether it was the medications, or what they did to her brain, I don't know. But slowly, slowly, she came back. We didn't discuss my father much. For the last 10 or 15 years she's been good, but I have dreaded this moment, when she became ill herself."

"Why do you think her own illness will trigger severe depression again. I mean, I'm not a psychiatrist, but if her depression stemmed from guilt, why should her own illness make her feel guilty?"

"It's a complicated business doctor. The mind doesn't work in such a linear way. But I was warned, that any major trauma could do it. And here we are. Here we are. It's started."

Nina looked down, at the tops of her shoes. She sighed. Then she looked up.

"I'm sorry Mr Lewis. There was no satisfactory way to do this. I'm sorry I didn't wait for you, but…in a way, it just had to be done. She knows the facts, and she will not be left on her own. You are here."

"If that makes you feel better, fine. Why did you tell her? You didn't know anything about her. It was…arrogant."

"I'm sorry."

And Nina knew that he was right, she should not have gone ahead. What was it? A sense of pressure, to progress the situation; an overly elevated perception of her own ability to communicate, to deal with emotionally situations; or an immature response to the interference of an absent relative, a message channelled through a ward nurse, telling her what not to do? Whatever the reason, she wished she had waited.

Agree not to tell Dorothy anything else without referring to her son first and refer to oncology, go to 7

Refuse to be constrained by son's demand, go to 21

20.

Nina watched Dorothy carefully for a couple of days. She dithered over the antibiotics, not sure whether they were doing anything useful or not. She was on the point of crossing all non-essential drugs off the drug chart, but hesitated because it wasn't entirely clear that she was truly 'end of life'. She wished the palliative care team were involved. Perhaps when Dorothy became unresponsive, and communication was clearly impossible, they would agree to attend.

"Hi Nina!" The pall care nurse stood at her side.

"Hi. I thought you weren't coming."

"Of course we are. The ward sister rang us. You've got yourself into a right pickle haven't you?"

"Yes, you could say that."

"Is she awake?"

"Yes, but barely."

"Come on, let's go and see her."

They approached Dorothy's bed. She was unconscious. The House Officer was trying to put a venflon in. He had already failed three times.

"What IV's is she on?" asked the pall care nurse.

"Tazocin."

"Does she really need it? Really? She looks very close to the end."

Nina looked at the bruises on her patient's arm, and saw how damaging the delay in actively managing her impending death had been.

Go to Summing Up

21.

"I'm sorry Mr Lewis, I can't agree to that."

"What are you saying. You'll ignore my concerns completely?"

"Of course not, you know her the best, your feelings about how she wants to be treated are very important…but…we must reach an agreement, or we cannot give her the care that she needs. Care requires communication, her understanding, her comments…otherwise we are interpreting everything through a filter, and we may be missing subtle things that she is not being the opportunity to express. I can't be constrained."

"But I am her next of kin, I have a right…"

"It's about her Mr Lewis, about what she needs right now."

Dorothy's son had a developed a steely expression. For once, Nina realised that she was not going to be able to resolve this. It didn't happen very often.

"So…" she said.

"So. You know what I think. I have warned you. You do as you must, but if you harm her…"

And he left.

Go to 8

22.

Nina watched, Nina waited. She kept the blood pressure up, arranged blood units, and felt increasingly comfortable with the situation. Perhaps the bleeding had slowed, or even stopped. Dorothy's son arrived. He joined them. He nodded at Nina. Nina spoke,

"Mrs Lewis. Before we take you down to deal with this bleeding I'd like you to know what exactly we are worried about. You do need to know." Dorothy mumbled, but Nina was not sure that she was engaged. Nina continued,

"Your liver can showed some abnormalities, lumps...of tissue that shouldn't be there. We are worried it might be cancer."

She wasn't listening. Nina grabbed her hand. It was cool, and the pulse was racing. The bleeding had accelerated.

"Can I have some help here," she called out, into the ward.

"She's bleeding, seriously. We've left it too late."

Nina kept her fingers on the pulse. Something changed. Her hand leapt to Dorothy's neck. No pulse. Dorothy was dead. Nina ran to the phone on nurses' station to put out a crash call. Then she hesitated. Was it appropriate? Was it right? So much had not been discussed, so much had been left unsaid. This was the most disastrous day of her life.

Go to Summing Up

23.

Nina called Dorothy's son. She asked him to come to the ward as soon as possible. She gave little away, and adopted an assertive tone. She could not let this situation drag on any further. Shortly, they sat in the relatives' room, with Dorothy's nurse taking a third chair. Nina began,

"What happened to Dorothy, with the depression?"

"She spent 6 months in an...institution. This was in the 1980's. She had electroconvulsive therapy, to bring her out of a catatonic state. They delved into her mind, traced it back to my father's diagnosis. After she came home – I was at university during this period – she was not the same. Whether it was the medications, or what they did to her brain, I don't know. But slowly, slowly, she came back. We didn't discuss my father much. For the last 10 or 15 years she's been good, but I have dreaded this moment, when she became ill herself."

"Why do you think her own illness will trigger severe depression again. I mean, I'm not a psychiatrist, but if her depression stemmed from guilt, why should her own illness make her feel guilty?"

"It's a complicated business doctor. The mind doesn't work in such a linear way. But I was warned, that any major trauma could do it. And here we are. Here we are. It's started."

Nina looked down, at the tops of her shoes. She sighed. Then she looked up.

"I'm sorry Mr Lewis. There was no satisfactory way to do this. But I must insist that she is told about the diagnosis. She is dying, and there are aspects of her care that cannot be given properly if she remains in the dark. And beyond that, don't you think she should have the opportunity to understand, to collect her thoughts, perhaps look back over her life and say goodbye, rather than slip into unconsciousness?"

"She will spend her final hours and days thinking about my father, dwelling on her own role in his drawn out death. It will be so damaging."

"You are assuming that will happen/ And even if it does, perhaps it is appropriate – I'm not being cruel – for her to be thinking about these things, and putting her life into some sort of order, mentally. And we must accept this, that she does have much time, and will not experience the type of psychological symptoms that she suffered before."

"You mean, her physical death will overtake her depression."

"I'm sure of it. Does that give you a different perspective?"

"It does."

"She needs to know. She probably knows already."

Dorothy's son stared up, into a corner of the room. When he regained his focus he nodded.

"OK. We'll do it together."

Go to Summing Up

24.

"Hello, Lisa. I need help. Things have got out of hand here with a patient."

Nina told the palliative care nurse everything.

"Yes, I see. That is a mess. Sounds like you need some support!"

"Well, I can face up to the conversation – with the patient or her son – but if she does disintegrate, or refuses to engage…then the bottom line is I have let things go on for too long. I know I should have dealt with it earlier…"

"Hey, don't cut yourself up. I'll come up to the ward. We are telling her. Now."

And they did.

Go to 11

Summing Up – Collusion

I think this scenario is less about having to decide *what* to do, and more about *why* the situation has come about. Nina is presented with an unwinnable set of choices, and only when she slows down and asks the patient's son why he thinks Dorothy would not want to be told about the cancer, does she learn about her 6 month internment in a psychiatric hospital (if you did not find these sections, the route is 1>2>5>19, or 1>4>6>8>10>12>24). This knowledge allows some sort of insight into the son's frame of mind. Some choices lead to a calm referral to palliative care, and it is this outcome that seems to be best that can be achieved.

The traps that are set in this case illustrate the dangers of avoiding the issue and colluding with the 'game' of protecting Dorothy from the truth: complications from a biopsy that she could not fully consent to, or rushed communications when she develops pneumonia, for instance. End of life decisions begin to be taken without the patient's opinion or feelings being taken into account – all this because the patient's likely feelings were anticipated and *presumed* at the outset. Dorothy's son forbade full disclosure, and his motives were good, but they had to be challenged by the medical team, because they knew that delay would tie them all up in knots.

I'm sure there are occasions when the decision to withhold information from patients with full mental capacity can be defended, but they must be rare. Such patients are usually deteriorating quickly, and there are few actual decisions to be made. Or perhaps they are not remembering the facts from one day to another , and it is felt that reiterating those facts every time you see the patient is not constructive.

What Nina did not have the opportunity to explore in this case was the son's own motivations. It is possible that the limits set by him represented his own fears for his own inability to cope, rather than his mother's inability to cope. Perhaps keeping her in the dark would save him some difficult conversations. Perhaps things happened in the family that he does not want to revisit, perhaps he harbours guilt about his own role in his father's death. Who knows? Human life is subtle, and sometimes things go unsaid. Doctors are not psychoanalysts, and can only delve so deep.

This open access BMJ article (2000), *'Collusion in doctor-patient communication about imminent death: an ethnographic study'* looks into collusion with patients (rather than relatives) on the matter of over-optimistic prognoses in lung cancer. *'Reducing Collusion Between Family Members and Clinicians of Patients Referred to the Palliative Care Team'* (2009) and *'Communication with Relatives and Collusion in Palliative Care: A Cross-Cultural Perspective'* (2009) discuss the issue in relation to different cultural backgrounds.

The patient as riddle

Recently a patient said to me, 'Thank you for taking an interest.' This compliment reveals a whole world of problems. It says, in ascending order of alarm –

- Up until now no-one has been interested
- I've been looking for someone to invest their time and attention in my problem
- …because until someone takes an interest in you, things don't get done
- …and if you don't manage to find a doctor who is interested in you, you're on your own
- Will anybody actually engage in my problem if I'm not *interesting*?

So what role does interest play in the patient-doctor relationship?

Sparks

A patient enters the clinic room. Another referral, another challenge. But the referral letter includes some tantalising pieces of information, and the patient describes how an unusual symptom developed three weeks after returning from, say, Bolivia. Sparks of interest meet the kindling of barely remembered lectures on tropical disease; you search your memory, plan some investigations. After clinic you make a special effort to expedite a scan or ensure that a special blood test is sent away to another lab. The game is afoot. The game? Is this really a game?

Doctors are problem solvers. There are many problems to solve in medicine, and until you qualify those problems are generally intellectual – a combination of pattern recognition when presented with pathology, and cross referencing disparate physical symptoms or signs with the huge database of information that has been created during your medical education. At his or her purest, the useful doctor is an inspired search engine, able to discard irrelevant diagnoses and focus on the probable, before seeking confirmatory data to back up the initial hunch. In training the focus is knowledge and its application. How many doctors reading this, as students, left a ward full of ill patients in a huff, muttering, 'No signs, no *signs!*'?

But the first day on the wards presents very different problems to solve, such as how to prioritise an unmanageable list of jobs, how to persuade a radiologist to perform a CT scan in the desired time frame, how to placate the nurse who needs you to re-write a drug chart while you run off to an emergency. A job that seemed cerebral becomes predominantly organisational, and this can make some young doctors downhearted. Then, if you persevere, learn how the system works and become more senior, the opportunity to make diagnoses and test hypotheses yourself comes around. You admit patients, see, hear and feel the signs that you once read about in books, and start to believe in medicine again! You begin to see 'interesting cases'.

The high priests

What advantage do 'interesting cases' have? By virtue of the clinical features that these patients report or display, they generate energy. They stimulate conversations, the swapping of ideas, the easing open of dusty books (or more, likely, tapping into PubMed), the seeking of multiple opinions…the chase is on to get the right answer and find the right treatment. While such focus is commendable, if not vital in some urgent cases, the price may come when doctors get carried away in the search for jigsaw pieces that fit the puzzle and lose sight of the person before them.

In '5 patients' (available to read for free here) the late Michael Crichton wrote about the game that can play out when a student or trainee and their supervisor spar over the meaning of various clues, and presented an impenetrable piece of dialogue as an example:

Student: "The patient has kidney disease consistent with glomerulonephritis."

Visit (by which he means a resident or attending, I think-PB): "Was there a recent history of infection?"

Student: "Anti-streptolysin titers were low."

63

Visit: "Was there a facial rash?"

Student: "LE prep and anti-nuclear antibodies were negative."

Visit: "Were there eye background changes?"

Student: "Glucose-tolerance test was normal."

Visit: "Did you consider rectal biopsy?"

Student: "The tongue was not enlarged."

The conversation 'jumps from mountain top to mountain top' as both parties demonstrate that they know what the other is referring to without saying what they mean explicitly. They are caught up in a trail of clues and deductions; if the patient were listening (as is often the case on ward rounds or teaching clinics), they would be bewildered. But patients do tend to tolerate such jargon heavy, exclusive exchanges, recognising that they are relevant to their own condition even if they are beyond their understand. In such scenarios paternalism, even sacerdotalism (whereby doctors act as mediators between humans and the unknowable mysteries of the body) rise again.

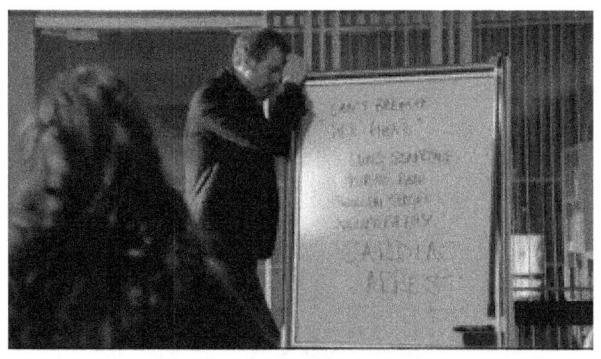

The whiteboard

A seductive game

As non-patients, we enjoy such games. Hence the popularity of TV shows like ER (created by Crichton) and House, where the plot is driven by a race against time to understand the relevance of various medical clues. Despite the human interest, the success of these shows depends on the writers' ability to find a good medical topic, be it radiation sickness or the clichéd 'lupus', and set up a sense of jeopardy. The famous whiteboard, on which House's photogenic team record their ideas, illustrates how medicine must, when pared down to its essentials, focus on the facts. The working title for House was 'Chasing zebras, circling the drain', zebras being rare conditions. House was itself inspired by the work of a New Yorker journalist, Berton Roueche, who wrote up real life cases of medical detection from 1940s until his death from suicide by shotgun in the 1990s. Eleven Blue Men (1953) presents 11 such cases, and is for sale in hardback on Amazon at £143! There is no doubt about it, doctors and non-doctors alike are fascinated by zebras.

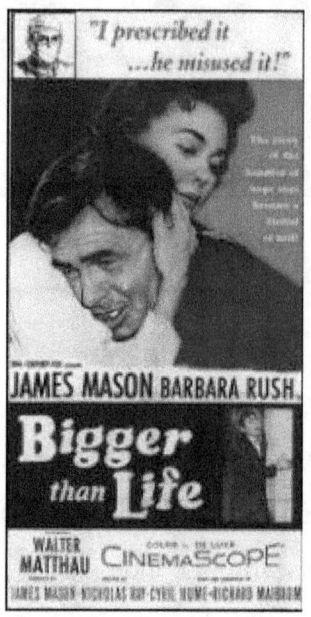

The film Bigger Than Life, starring James Mason as a patient with polyarteritis nodosa who becomes addicted to cortisone, is based on Berton Roueche's work.

It and Thou

Back in the real world the physician <u>Jeffrey Ennis explored this progression</u> from the factual to the holistic explored by reflecting on his own experiences. He presented to hospital with neurological symptoms such as shoulder pain and tongue numbness, which were eventually diagnosed as due to Guillain-Barre syndrome. He contrasted the attitude of the emergency physician, which he found 'insensitive and depersonalizing' with that of the neurologist, who was 'comforting'. Ennis then invoked the philosopher Martin Buber's categories of 'I-It' and 'I-Thou' relationships, and concluded his piece with this:

'The physician-patient relationship is the vehicle through which such care is provided. In an I-It relationship, the patient and the problem are objectified, allowing the physician to collect and analyze data about the patient's problem in an effort to offer a solution. Taken to an extreme, an I-It relationship can be dehumanizing.

At the other end of the spectrum of human interaction is the I-Thou relationship, where the physician experiences the patient as an emotional being. This allows the clinician to empathize with the individual's situation and to offer psychological support. Taken to an extreme an I-Thou relationship can result in the clinician becoming confluent with the patient's emotional state. As a result of this, the physician becomes psychologically paralyzed and is unable to offer objective clinical assistance to the patient.'

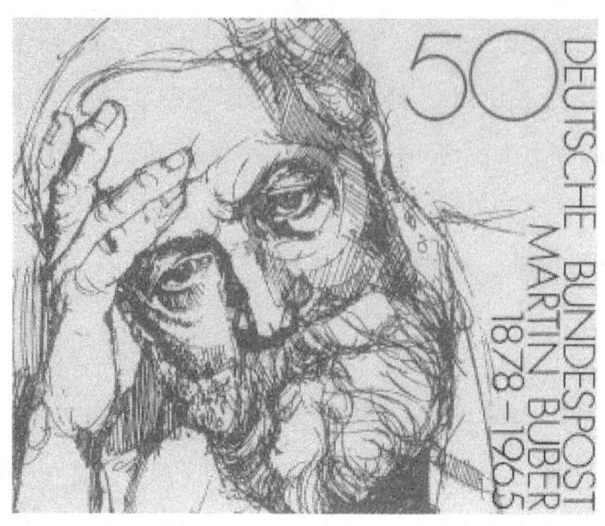

Martin Buber, philosopher

There is clearly a place for both, but they lie on a spectrum. In my mind the balance tips towards the I-It in emergency situations, where the jeopardy is greatest and the unknowns are numerous. Then, having achieved a degree of safety and stability, the doctor can move towards the I-Thou end of the spectrum. This approach might seem reasonable, but…it fails. It fails because patients are at their most distressed and vulnerable during that early period of uncertainty, and it is at this time that they need to see human qualities and a willingness to empathise. Traditionally, nurses have been better at recognising psychological distress in emergency situations, and have been able to compensate for doctors' tunnelled medical vision. However, as doctors, the ability to retain an awareness of the whole patient rather than the just the relevant physical features can soften a potentially petrifying experience. Away from severe emergencies, the ability to keep an eye on the Thou without letting the clues in the It slip through unnoticed remains an important medical skill. Melding the two – forensic analysis and human warmth, always was a tall order.

The essence of satisfaction

Most conditions and presentations are easily recognisable and do not excite a fascinated reaction or the doctor to go to the textbooks. It is not acceptable for this majority to perceive themselves as boring in the eyes of their doctors. To each patient their own ailment is of paramount interest, and the doctor who fails to reflect a sense of uniqueness will come across badly. But for those doctors who derive genuine professional pleasure only from the interesting patients, a career in which the majority are *not* interesting may prove challenging. How to resolve this?

My advice would be - do your best to work in a field that you find interesting and enjoy the 'game' when you are required to play it. However, no specialty or department that I know of is exclusively populated by patients who succeed in creating those intellectual sparks. If it doesn't come naturally, it behoves doctors to develop ways of deriving interest from patients in a way that does not rely solely on their medical condition. The rewards of making the right diagnosis are fleeting, because once made the process of arriving at it becomes irrelevant. It is treatment and management, which may be long term for chronic conditions (such as lupus, for example!), or barely effective in others, that really matters. Moreover, it is the patient's wellbeing as a whole person, not a collection of affected organs, that is the true measure success. If we as doctors are not 'interested' in that, ultimate satisfaction will be denied.

Singular histories, common needs:
replacing the LCP

The Leadership Alliance for the Care of Dying People published its interim report just as I was beginning to wonder what had become of the urgent changes set into motion by Baroness Neuberger's report on the Liverpool Care Pathway. Those of us outside the specialist palliative care community but deeply involved in the care of the dying (i.e. nurses, hospital specialists and general practitioners) are not privy to the day to day developments behind the scenes. Since the LCP was withdrawn, its commendable intentions besmirched by association with CQUIN payments and isolated poor practice, patients have continued to die. We presume, we hope, that they have died in as much comfort, and with as much dignity, that health care professionals were able to provide.

The conclusions of the Leadership Alliance have been anticipated to some degree. Prominent critics of the LCP fear that the current exercise is no more than 'rebranding'. Professor Pullicino, whose presentation to the Medical Ethics Alliance in large part set the ball rolling, has been quoted as saying,

"The fact is that little seems to have changed, including the use of syringe drivers, anticipatory prescribing, use of sedation and narcotics and limitation of hydration and nutrition by a 'best interest' team decision." The Neuberger report accepted that these aspects of care had an important place in palliation, so it seems extremely unlikely that the Professor's suspicious attitude to them will percolate into the Leadership Alliance's proposals.

Not missed

Do I miss the LCP? Strangely, for one who regretted its withdrawal, the answer is no. I realised this a few months after the Neuberger report was published (by which time many trusts had stopped using it), and had to ask myself why. My conclusion – effective protocols make work* for those who follow them, and when any protocol or treatment pathway is withdrawn, other business rapidly fills the space. The LCP committed clinicians to a degree of engagement with the needs of dying patients, and its sudden absence (without a replacement) may allow those caring for patients to move along more swiftly to the next. I have no evidence that care for the dying has suffered since the LCP was withdrawn, but know that I, personally, am spending less time on the little things. This may be for want of structure. The LCP, with its spaces for daily nursing and medical entries, with its reminders to check those aspects of bodily comfort that might otherwise be overlooked, served to draw us into the dying patient's passive sphere. The pathway imposed on us, but ensured that we dedicated the time that was required to maximise comfort. In its absence we have the fundamental aspects of palliative care (which are not complicated, after all) to guide us, and in many Trusts some bridging guidance or condition specific approaches have been developed, but we do not have an instantly recognisable, well rehearsed approach. There is much to be said for the common language and mutual understanding that the LCP generated between doctors and nurses.

The semantics of protocols and pathways

What was the LCP? According to Neuberger,

'The LCP provides alerts, guidance and a structured, single record for doctors, nurses and multidisciplinary teams that are inexpert in palliative care.'

However, it seemed to become more than that – a deterministic force,

'...the LCP is being perceived by some of its users – doctors and nurses – not as a document, nor as a guideline, but most frequently as a set of instructions and prescriptions, that is to say a protocol.'

The authors then explore the concept of the pathway, differentiating between various different forms of guidance. As someone who uses all of these types of document on a weekly basis, I nevertheless find the following paragraph quite a handful -

'To remove this lack of clarity and the unintended consequences that appear to follow from it, the Review panel recommends that NHS England and NICE should review urgently the terms they are using to define clinical 'pathways', distinguishing them from protocols, standard operating procedures, guidelines, guidance, and best practice models. These must be intelligible to all, from clinicians to members of the public.'

The principles on which new guidelines will be based emphasise the importance of asking, listening and tailoring care to the expressed wishes of the patient and family. But we will need some sort of 'protocol' to encompass those principles and *remind* us, if not *compel* us, to apply them. Is it possible to do that without paper, a checklist...a booklet? The Leadership Alliance states in its interim document that it will be producing a 'prompt sheet'. It is accepted that we, the doctors and nurses at the front line, *need* to be reminded.

The problem of inexorability

What differentiates a pathway from a protocol? To me, pathway suggests a sense of the inexorable, and it is that, in this context, which causes concern. For once patients had been started on a pathway,

'Many patients and their families felt as though they have lost control over what was happening to them.'

74

The following extract from the report touches on this sense of inevitability,

'A repeated observation by families was that starting the LCP seemed to mean that proper clinical assessments of the need for medication ceased, instead of occurring every four hours as recommended in the LCP document; the LCP was then experienced as if it were a protocol, even a "tick-box" exercise, through which the next step was to stop food and fluids and give continuous infusions of strong opioids and sedatives without justification or explanation.'

It is the lack of transparency or sharing of thoughts that causes most concern. We can, I think, be reasonably sure that doctors and nurses *were* thinking, but perhaps, with a sense of justification permitted by the acceptance of inevitable decline on the pathway, health care workers did not see the need to explain and discuss. The LCP foresaw such developments and accounted for them, but it may have short-circuited the need to share and re-confirm, with families, that they were comfortable with developments. Neuberger highlights the shock felt by families when patients were found unable to converse just a few hours after appearing alert,

'There have been too many people coming forward to the Review panel to state that they left their loved one in a calm and peaceful state, able to communicate, for a short time, or with a doctor or nurse for a check-up, only to return to find a syringe driver had been

put in place and their loved one was never able to communicate again. ...the Review panel felt that patients, their relatives and carers should be told the reasons for "step changes" in treatment, and be given the opportunity to contribute to a discussion about appropriate care.'

To nurses and doctors, such changes are part of dying, and not necessarily a reason to make a new telephone call; to the family, such changes are full of meaning.

Finding the singular in the ubiquitous

Which brings me to the concept of individualised care. This, to me, is the paradox that must somehow be overcome by those responsible for replacing the LCP. How do we ensure that common management principles are universally and strictly applied by variously trained doctors and nurses, while maintaining the sense of bespoke care?

The more I consider the demise of the LCP, the more I focus on the possibility that we, the medical profession, misjudged the significance of death's sanctity in the eyes of our patients' relatives. I do not refer to religious sanctity, but the oneness, the singularity of each life as it slips into death. I am increasingly convinced that the normal expectations of consensus between doctor and patient (or doctor and relative) do not apply in end of life scenarios. Perhaps my experience is skewed to those rapidly progressive conditions and unexpected deteriorations that occur on general medical wards, but there is something uncomfortable about meeting this situation with a *prepared* approach that one can extract from the filing cabinet behind the nurses' station. The impression it gives is, 'Oh yes, we have a process for that.'

However sensitive the clinician, however skilful their communication, any sense of individualisation is likely to be negated by the perception that common rules are being applied. Some relatives say as much, for example, 'I'm sure you see this all the time doctor…but I haven't lost a parent before.'

We, as clinicians, have indeed seen it all before, and even those of us who have been bereaved will be in 'work mode', where death is commonplace and everything has its place in a ward filled with illness and anxiety.

Every death is unique. Few would disagree with that. But doctors and nurses, who have observed death many times, will say that there is much in common between them. What makes each death unique is the life leading up to it. That life is initially invisible to medical staff. For families, death is the culmination of a rich experience. For those providing care, who can only guess at the depth of their patient's history, death is the end result of disease. As layers of personality and snippets of history are added to the initial sketch, the true meaning of *this* death becomes clear. This difference of perception - the rich, full person as perceived by the family on the one hand, the unremarkable process of dying common to all terminal patients as perceived by medical staff on the other, may explain the problems that have arisen around the LCP.

The onward flow

The flattening effects of such philosophical and emotional influences are further exaggerated by the pressured atmosphere of a busy ward; an inadequate relatives' room, bleeps that have not been deactivated during preparation for a crucial conversation, noisy vacuum cleaners. The quotidian, unremarkable nature of death is impressed on families, and the Neuberger report included examples to reinforce this picture of 'business as usual', such as,

'Privacy screens were normally open so that all visitors, cleaning staff and the other patients could witness my uncle's distress and imminent demise.'

or,

'Catering staff asking quite loudly in the middle of the ward to other patients what food and drink they would like is completely inappropriate when my uncle was under the LCP.'

The challenge of remaining sensitive to the unique aspects of each patient, their history, their preferences, their relatives' expectations, while ensuring that needs common to all dying people are not overlooked, remains huge. I don't envy the Leadership Alliance in the task of preserving all that was good in the LCP while designing something fundamentally different.

oOo

* I explored the idea of LCP as 'work' in a previous post 'An opaque code: the Liverpool Care Pathway and a gap in perception'

Making deals: the problem of the self
discharging patient

There are times when a patient's dissatisfaction stretches the therapeutic relationship to its limits. Take this example – a man of 32 survives an eight day admission on the intensive care unit, for, say, pneumonia. He is discharged to the ward, but develops a pneumothorax – a collapsed lung. In the middle of the night a chest drain is inserted, he improves, and the following day his team come to see him on a ward round. The drain is out. What happened?

"I sat on it…the tubing." This happens.

"OK, we'll arrange for another one to be inserted this morning."

"I don't need one. I'm going home today." Of course, the clue was there – he has dressed himself in his usual clothes.

"Well, John, that's a bit premature. You're lung could collapse down again at any time. We were advised to keep that drain in for a few days at least, to make sure it wasn't still leaking."

"I'm fine. Listen to my lungs." He lifts up the front of his shirt.

"I will, in a moment, but let's just agree on today shall we. You will stay, won't you?"

"No. I'm going. I've already called my mate, he's picking me up during his lunch hour."

"We can't...look John, if you go home there's a good chance your lung will collapse and you'll be as ill as you were overnight. It wasn't good, was it?"

"It's not going to happen again. You can't tell me it is. Doctor, I've been very reasonable...very patient, with everything you've asked me..."

And so it starts. The suggestion, that we, the doctors, have somehow imposed on him.

"...I let you put me to sleep, go on the ventilator...two weeks I've lost, I've got people I need to see, things to do..."

As though the decisions we made were to inconvenience him...

"But I'm better now. They said on intensive care that the infection has gone, someone my age can get better a lot faster than...some of the old blokes you've got in here..."

"They were right. But it's not safe at the moment. If it does collapse, you'll be just as ill, if not sicker, than you were..."

And undo all the work that we have done!

"I'm grateful doctor. But I'm going. Today."

What next?

I have heard all of the following categories of response in this type of situation. Some sound wrong, but are understandable; some are morally right but medically unsafe. Which would you choose?

A. *"This is a hospital, not a prison..."* The classic riposte. It's true of course, treatment is entirely voluntary, and a patient, having been informed about the risks, has the perfect right to walk away. To me this response (which, I'll admit, I have been driven to use) represents a complete breakdown of the physician-patient relationship. It is a surrender, to the complexity of the challenge. You might as well say what you're thinking, which is 'Fine, I'm *DONE* with you!'

How does this conversation end? Often, with this – "But you will need to sign a self-discharge form." This may crystallise, in the mind of the patient, the fact that responsibility for what happens to them from that point on is all theirs. It is a form a brinkmanship, watching to see if they change their mind as they write their name. Brinkmanship really has no place in good medicine.

B – *"We'll let you go...but you must understand, if you do deteriorate your bed will be gone, you'll need to call an ambulance and come to A and E..."* The blackmail. By describing how difficult it will be to re-engage with the hospital you hope to dissuade him. You avoid invoking the emotional angle, emphasising how disappointed you are that all the 'hard work will be undone', but the loss of 'the bed' signifies this. The bed is the symbol of the care that they have received, and by losing it to another patient they sacrifice the therapeutic bond that duty and need forged between you.

John's departure will be semi-condoned, so as not to require a self-discharge letter. But this is risky, from the point of view of the doctors, for if John *does* collapse and die on the high street, the medical team will have no documentation with which to defend themselves. By maintaining a relationship they open themselves up to criticism.

C – *"I understand John, I'd want to go if I was in your position. But give us 24, 48 hours...please. That's all we need. Then we'll get you home, I promise."* The bargain. A false one at that, because you have no idea what the next day or two will hold. He may require another chest drain, or worse, transfer to a cardio-thoracic unit... it's a lie (albeit well intentioned) to promise anything in medicine. You have paid for his compliance by making a commitment that you may not be able to fulfil. The push back, in two days, may be all the more intense.

D – *"I understand John, I'd want to go if I was in your position. Let's see what we can work out."* And you go on to explore a true compromise. He goes home, but you arrange for him to come up to the ward every day for a quick check over; or for the SHO to call him, to make sure he is still breathing well; or for the GP to do the same. A truly personalised approach. It sounds like good medicine – it takes into account his specific concerns, his anxiety to get back to work, his need for freedom!

But is it realistic? By making these arrangements you create extra work and unusual demands on your team, or the GP. John needs to be monitored or he does not; and if he *does*, he needs to be in hospital. Simple as. What sounds and feels reasonable may actually be unreasonable, even if it does maintain the therapeutic relationship.

E – *"I understand that you need to leave. But let's think about this…let's put it into perspective."* Thus speaks the philosopher. You go on to explain, 'John. If you don't make a full recovery from this you could be in and out of hospital for weeks, months. If you can just spend some time focussing on your health now, even it takes longer than you'd like, you can get better properly and avoid longer term problems. Then, a year from now, looking back on this time it will be just a blip…you'll be back at work, with it all behind you." Such subtle mind-tricks can work, because they are, in fairness, reasonable. Patients who cannot accept their ill health, who continuously resist management plans that will entail longer periods of hospitalisation, might benefit from the odd dose of perspective.

The danger, from the doctor's point of view, is that of sounding patronising. After all, it's not you who are away from work and family for weeks on end. The problem with this approach is that it doesn't change a thing, materially.

Finally, there is the approach that fewer doctors, in busy wards, confronted by aggression or apparent ingratitude, will take; that of sitting down, ignoring the rush of oncoming clinical traffic, and exploring what it is, really, that troubles the patient. For there is bound to be a source of stress, be it financial, inter-personal or domestic that can be identified and addressed. Perhaps it's an addiction; perhaps it's their turn to look after the kids this weekend. To find out what it is requires an ability to ignore the simmering anger, and to understand the emotional heat created when illness afflicts younger generations who are use to running their own lives quite satisfactorily in normal circumstances. A tall order, that only the most disciplined can succeed in – and on a good day at that.

Tempting fate: the perils of reassurance

A patient comes to the clinic with common enough symptoms – say a slight change in bowel habit and a single episode of bleeding. It could be a cough that doesn't go away, or a lump in the groin, or a pain in the back that doesn't settle – but something about it has led the GP to refer on to a specialist. By the time he sees you the bowels have gone back to normal and the bleeding has settled. You examine him – all is well, but nevertheless you explain that the only way to exclude anything dangerous is to do a colonoscopy. But he is anxious, and presses you.

"Do you think it's anything serious doctor?"

"We need to wait for the camera test. It's impossible to say without looking inside."

"But what do you think doctor? Honestly."

"I wouldn't want to second guess the test."

"Well you must be worried if you think I need it."

"Your symptoms are a bit worrying, as your GP explained to you. And there's no escaping the fact that the main reason we arrange colonoscopies in these situations is to exclude serious diseases, like cancer."

"But you don't think…"

"I don't want you to be worrying excessively over the next few weeks Mr. Evans. But I can't rule it out."

"Oh God."

"Look. If you pressed me, I'd say that the fact that you haven't had any bleeding or loose stools for 6 weeks, and your normal blood tests…suggest you're probably OK. Lots of people get symptoms like yours and in the end we find nothing. But we must wait. Sorry."

"That's OK doctor. I feel better now."

And two weeks later you see him again. You have already been informed that the colonoscopy found a cancer. Mr Evans had a staging CT scan yesterday, and there are suspicious lesions in the liver. It's terrible news, although, in an era of highly effective chemotherapy and adventurous liver surgery, not necessarily a terminal diagnosis. He looks at you rather coldly. The hopes that you allowed him to develop, leading up to the colonoscopy, have been brutally dashed. You discuss options, plans, schedules...

Was it a mistake to proffer an opinion? Isn't that what doctors are for? Nine times out of 10 your impression, your gut feeling as to the seriousness of the diagnosis, would be right; perhaps more than that, probably 99 out a 100. And by giving some encouragement, albeit with caveats, you ensure that many patients suffer less anxiety, or spend less time in unhealthy pre-occupation with their impending tests and results. And in 99 cases out of a 100 that encouragement proves well founded, until...you get it wrong. Then it feels as though you have misled the less fortunate patient - colluded in their natural wish to see the bright side, contributed to the trauma of the sudden, more precipitous fall.

After one of these experiences, you will be more guarded. For the next 6 months, the next year, you will maintain an inscrutable front, until, having received numerous negative test reports, you dare once again to reassure an anxious patient who comes with seemingly innocent complaints.

- - -

Sweet Hope, celestial influence round me shed
Waving thy silver pinions o'er my head.
Keats, To Hope, February 1815

Students, you make us better doctors

As a medical student, I remember a consultant saying to me, "Watch what I do, take away what you like, forget what you don't. Do that throughout your career and you'll end up emulating the best of your trainers." I found this strange, as it encouraged me to scrutinise the way senior doctors behaved. Now, as a consultant, I recognise that whatever I say or do is considered and judged by those I train.

This creates a pressure, to put across the best of myself. And that requires energy. So, if I walk into a clinic room and am told by the nurse that there is a student waiting for me, I may experience a brief "Oh...really?" Many students will have witnessed a slight deflation in the faces of doctors to whom they have been attached for the morning or afternoon - as though to say, "What a pain!" Their presence will change the way I conduct myself. I will have to be mindful of their need to understand and be involved with the consultations (otherwise they will become completely bored). And it will complicate my interaction with patients, should they appear hesitant or show signs of annoyance when I introduce the observer. What would have been a series of two-way interactions turns into a three way, dual purpose conversation. All of this requires an investment of concentration and effort.

This apparent downside has advantages. Having accepted the fact that I have a student, I will move into a different gear. I become teacher and doctor. My behaviour tends to improve. If I find myself behaving less than perfectly, I will remind myself that the impression I am making is contributing to the development of that young student or doctor. They will either accept or reject my approach, not formally, not such that their impression will be fed back to me, but cumulatively. I do not want them to look back, four years hence, and say, "Yes I remember seeing a consultant do such and such, and I told myself there and then that I never wanted to be like that with patients." (We all have examples we can think of, I'm sure!) We only have to look back on our own evolution as students, junior doctors and middle grades, to recognise that the way we behave now is due to an accumulation of different experiences and different judgments. None of us want to display behaviours that end up on the discarded pile.

What else does the student bring to the clinic or ward? He or she brings the need for clarity. Their questions have a habit of cutting through any pretence to omniscience that we may have maintained while trying to understand a complicated concept or disease. Just as a fallible maths teacher may crumble in the face of an apparently naive question about geometry from a 10 year old, so a medical student's simple enquiry about auto-antibodies or cardiac murmurs can reveal the true depth of one's true understanding. To avoid such discomfiture in the future, you may even go and look it up for first time in ten years. Sometimes, you find yourself explaining a complex situation to the patient and the student simultaneously. This generates a true sense of engagement, and can result in a successful scientific or technical interpretation, understood by both in plain language.

They can also work, quietly, to preserve our humanity, and perhaps such a simple quality as politeness. If I'm running late, it is easy to fall into a pattern of hasty turnarounds and compressed consultations. Any temptation to hurry the patient along will be countered by the knowledge that efficiency tricks and verbal ticks are being observed. I may know the patient has unanswered questions, which I 'just do not have time' to address. One look at the student's face will tell me if I've been too hasty. Caught up in the ever-present temptation to hurry, the outsider's expression serves as a barometer of decency.

Perhaps some doctors, supremely confident in the way they behave, are not influenced by the presence of students. Others may put on a performance, energised by the showmanship that expertise and hierarchy can encourage..although this can result in the patient being excluded from the interaction. It has to be remembered that the axis of primary importance in the room is that between patient and doctor, not doctor and student.

So having students around can be a good thing, for patients. And for senior doctors they are valuable too, as moving mirrors, passing influencers, potent in their ability to reflect back the best and worst of our ingrained medical habits. Saying that, I would not want to be followed by students all hours, all days. Because they require attention, they will necessarily slow down whatever medical process they happen to be observing. Sometimes it is nice just to get on with your own thing, in your own way, even if that does involve falling back into your own bad habits (or catching up on emails). But now and again it does no harm at all for someone to put a mirror in the corner. Sometimes that mirror will speak, and, venturing outside the comfort zone of silence, say 'I thought you did that really well.'

The good in him

This post was inspired by the paper 'Culture, compassion and clinical neglect: probity in the NHS after Mid Staffordshire' (Journal of Medical Ethics, £) by Newdick and Danbury, in which the reasons why doctors appear as reluctant now as they ever were to report poor practice, are explored.

As ever in these fictions, I try to examine at a micro-psychological level, why doctors behave as they do. I do not presume to present a full or validated explanation.

oOo

Dev had always taken an interest in wider aspects of medicine; he had enjoyed epidemiology and public health modules at med school, he was tempted by the new focus on leadership in medicine, he looked at systems and wondered how things could be done better. After the Francis report, he asked himself, 'What will I do if I see poor or uncompassionate practice?' He did not know the answer to this, but knew that he would not ignore it if there were persistent or egregious examples. After all, hadn't he read that *'between 120 to 150 doctors must have known something was going badly wrong at*

Stafford Hospital yet few raised concerns through the proper channels'

A few weeks after starting work as a Foundation Year doctor he became aware of a particularly uncaring nurse. She was abrupt with the confused patients, and scolded them occasionally. It was shocking to hear, but no-one else seemed to notice. Her manner did prove effective, as those she admonished tended to settle down and desist (for that shift, anyway). Dev was aware of no complaints, but, mindful of recent lessons learnt, promised to stay alert and take the uncomfortable step of reporting her, to someone, if things got worse. He would start by discussing it with his registrar. Perhaps today. He and the registrar had just completed a ward round, and Dev was being given his directions for the day.

"So that's your mission. Get Mrs Wilkinson transferred. She's been waiting over a week, the bed managers are on our backs, she's getting tetchy. Spend a while getting the story straight in your own head, try to get through to the receiving team's registrar and explain why he, or she, needs to expedite things at their end."

"I'll try. There's lots to do for the other patients too."

"That's the trouble, we always have sicker patients to focus on and no-one has the time to devote their energies to situations like this. But today, let's do it. I'm in clinic, but call me if they give you any grief."

The registrar left, leaving Dev to contemplate tactics. It wasn't such a bad day really, the in-patients weren't too sick, there weren't too many outliers. He walked into Mrs Wilkinson's bay and touched her on the shoulder, waking her up.

"Mrs Wilkinson, it's Dev, the doctor. Just to say, we're going to pull out the stops today, try and get the transfer sorted."

"I'd be so grateful. I know it's not your fault, but I've been achieving nothing for the last week.

I'm worried I'm going to have another attack before I get there, and be too unwell for them..."

"I'll do my best."

As Dev left the ward his consultant was walking in; she took him to one side.

"Dev, I'm sorry, but we've been singled out for being so efficient! Two clerking SHO's have called in sick and they're short down in the AMU. I had to put my hand up and say we were pretty much under control...and I volunteered you for a shift. Can you stay a bit over today, as the clerking shift runs to 8PM. And come in late tomorrow. OK?"

"Errr...OK, fine. Mike asked me to get something done urgently, might take an hour..."

"I'm sure that's OK. If you could get down there by 11."

Dev called the tertiary team. The necessary scans had not come through, so they had not been reviewed – hence the delay in the transfer. Dev was told to get them across straight away. He didn't know how, but he would find out.

In radiology he waited patiently for an administrative assistant to come off the phone. The hospital to which they were referring Mrs W was not part of the usual network; the scans would need to be burned onto a disc and sent in the post.

"No way. That's not acceptable I'm afraid. Can't they be couriered?"

"We don't do that here. Your department will need to arrange that." Dev began to bristle. A familiar feeling of frustration began to build. The assistant told him in more detail what he needed to do. Two signatures, on a special form. His consultant, and the department manager...And the forms? We have them down here!

"Thanks. Will you burn the disc now?"

"I've got a load to do...look at this pile of requests!"

"Mine's urgent."

"They're all urgent young man."

The assistant left her desk to fetch him the form. Dev took his own request from the bottom of the pile and slipped it in higher up. He recognised the writing on one of those he had demoted; it belonged to a housemate.

Getting the scans away was just the first step. He would then have to tell the tertiary team that they were on the way, encourage them to seek the package, upload the discs, make a clinical decision, and get back to Dev with their final determination. His bleep went off.

"When can you get to AMU Dev?" It was the on-call registrar, who had been given his name as a volunteer.

"Soon. Soon."

He plotted a course through the hospital: consultant's office (or was she in clinic?), manager's suite on the eight floor, back to x-ray to pick up the disc, then the post room, where, he assumed, couriers were arranged once all the paperwork was complete.

Dev began to run. He laughed at himself - it's not even a crash call...it's a package!

In the stairwell a physiotherapist was taking a stroke patient up a few steps. Dev waited patiently for space to appear by their side, and when it did he leapt forward, with precision. But three floors up he encountered the same situation. He waited again, then jumped forward. The toe of his trailing shoe clipped the patient's walking frame, and knocked it from the step. The physio compensated, taking the patient's full weight.

"I'm so sorry!" said Dev.

"Careful!" she retorted.

Dev collected the first signature, then ran down up a further two floors. Three people stood at a turn, blocking it, doing nothing. Dev paused, excused himself, excused himself again, then nudged past. One of them looked up. Dev saw that he was holding a map of the Trust, labelled in Hindi. Dev knew the language, but he looked through the paper, into neutral space, pretending not to have perceived the truth of the situation - that this family were lost. He ran on. Still so much to do. He obtained the second signature, the package itself, and by ten past eleven the slim parcel was waiting for the motorcycle courier. He rang the registrar in London, and was told to ring back at 4.45PM exactly. Later, and the registrar would be in the afternoon round-up meeting.

The welcome Dev received in AMU was effusive.

At 4.40PM the alarm on his smartphone reminded him to extricate himself and get to a Trust phone. As he walked through the AMU, busy now, always busy at this hour, a patient called out to him. It was 4.42PM. Dev approached the bed space. An old man leaned forward, confused but distressed.

"Water." he asked. There was water on his bedside table.

"Water." He had water. But he needed someone to put it to his lips. 4.44PM. "I'll tell the nurse."

He got to the nurses' station. The phone was being used by another doctor. At 4.45PM it became free. Dev grabbed it. A nurse moved behind him, and Dev turned to alert her to the patient's need for water. The operator of the other hospital spoke, and Dev focussed on the main task of the day – the transfer. As he waited for the registrar to respond to the bleep, Dev saw, through a glass partition, the family of the thirsty patient arrive. He watched as they fussed over their father and exchanged unhappy looks. Dev turned his back to it, embarrassed by his small omission.

It all worked out. Mrs Wilkinson's case was discussed in the round-up meeting, and her transfer was agreed for the following day.

That evening four families shared their experiences.

An Asian family spoke about the rude doctor who ignored them on the stairs. It's the little things like that, the father explained, that make a hospital's reputation. A physiotherapist, over her pint, talked about one of the good looking House Officers who was getting too self-important nowadays. He has been quite kind when he started, she recalled.

The son and daughter of a very elderly man asked how it was, in this day and age, that a thirsty patient could wait forty-five minutes before being given a drink. They had found him desperate, parched, and had held the cup and straw to his grateful lips on their arrival. And Mrs Wilkinson, when her relatives arrived, described how Dr Dev had taken it upon himself to make all the arrangements, how he had refused to let it slip any further, how 'personal' didn't even come close, and how nothing could beat the NHS.

When Dev next saw the impatient, seemingly uncompassionate nurse, he watched her work. She was working hard. He didn't much like her manner, and knew that someone needed to have a word, but he looked back on some aspects of his own behaviour the previous day, and thought – 'Who am I to criticise?'

oOo

* referenced in the Newdick and Danbury paper, from 'Annual Accountability Hearing with the General Medical Council. London, House of Commons Health Committee, HC 1429, Session 2010–12: para 42'

Frigidarium: on post-mortems, and taking the plunge

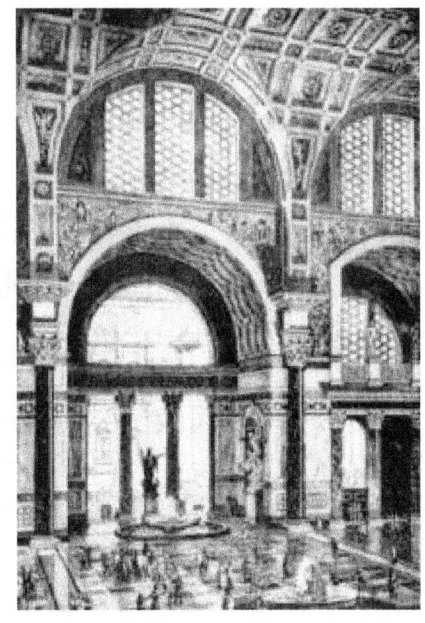

Frigidarium of the Baths of Caracalla, Rome (built 212-216)

[from Wikepedia]

The history of medicine is starred with single-minded men and women who were not afraid to look into the cold bodies of those whom they had failed to save. They did their best, but saw the post-mortem as a final duty. Thus they learnt what went wrong, and moved on to the next patient with greater understanding . In the modern era, pioneers have had no hesitation in dissecting patients whom they have come to know well, in order to learn – the case of Philip Blaiberg comes to mind, the second person to receive a heart transplant performed by Christiaan Barnard (19 months after surgery, his coronary arteries showed widespread atherosclerosis, now recognised as a feature of chronic rejection). It seems unthinkable that such a patient would *not* have a PM.

There are two types of post mortem: those performed by coroners and those requested by hospital doctors. Coroners remain active (more so since Shipman) and regularly take on cases where there is uncertainty as to the cause of death, but their focus is forensic and not inquisitive. The results of their investigations are not routinely fed back to medical teams, and they do not have the time or the resources to approach corpses with broad-minded medical curiosity.

As doctors we can still arrange hospital PMs if we wish, but we rarely do (personal observation). Since the organ retention scandal at Alder Hey the consent process has become far more demanding, and the consent form for relatives is very detailed (if not downright harrowing). Bureaucracy and nervousness are possible explanations for the rarity of hospital PMs, but I wonder if there is more to it.

Speaking for myself, there is a stark contrast between the memory of a patient and the idea of their supine form giving up its secrets to the gloved hands of the pathologist. It is not mere squeamishness, but is,

I believe, a more complex challenge. The cold plunge, from conversation one day to coarse incision the next, is shocking. Surely, the critic says, you are duty-bound to disregard such an emotional reaction, you must *try* to discover what happened. The 18th century, frock-coated and thick skinned physician in me thinks 'Yes'... but the modern doctor, the one who reassured the patient on day 1 that they were looking at no more than a week in hospital, and who on day 3 began to talk about discharge dates, thinks 'Wait... what good will it do him now?' The sudden transfer from concern for the individual to the 'greater good' is too turbulent, too cold.

The emphasis in modern healthcare is, quite rightly, compassion, and this requires empathy - a form of connection. It encourages a move away from regarding the patient as a mere body, or a dynamic data set. There is emotional engagement. So when our patients die unexpectedly we experience shock, there is a compressed form of grief, there may be a hint of guilt...and while these muddy waters swirl across the scene, a question looms – 'Shall we get a PM?' Perhaps, sometimes, we need to regain some of that old fashioned, hard-headed hunger for answers, in order to catch the truth before it disappears forever. It is no easy task.

Messengers

In hospital medicine, long term relationships with patients are rarer than one might expect. During training (which lasts until your mid-30's, and even longer for those who prevaricate!) it is unusual to stay in one Trust for more than a year. Becoming a consultant allows such relationships to develop, and this adds a depth of understanding and reward that cannot be experienced as a trainee. These are with patients who have chronic conditions, who attend clinic regularly, and who are occasionally admitted to the ward with complications; they comprise a small number compared to the thousands of 'one time only' interactions that take place each year. The irony is that while familiarity leads to trust and sincerity borne of shared experience, it is the fresh, short term clinical contacts that present the gravest clinical and emotional challenges. In these circumstances doctors must learn how to fast-track the communication strategies that will have already developed when meeting a long term patient. The classic example is talking to the patient with a new diagnosis of cancer.

In my mind breaking bad news follows a U shaped dynamic; constructive, forward planning allows the patient to be lifted from the despondency into which the word 'cancer' will have dragged them. By talking about what *can* be done, who they are likely to meet, resources and timescales...glimmers of hope may begin to permeate the gloom, and the certainty of death is diluted. The presence, ideally, of a cancer nurse specialist, reassures them that there will be continuity and reciprocal contact. Together we talk about the support that will be available, and the priority that will be given to their case.

But it is here that the limited nature of my role as 'first contact' begins to become clear. For however empathic my style, and however embracing my words, I know that *I* will have very little do with what happens from now on. As the patient (and family members, if present) look at me and the intensity of the situation burns its way into their memory, I know that it is not my face that they will be seeing in clinic. It will be that of the oncologist, or the surgeon (should the tumour prove operable). Already I am beginning to deflect responsibility to others – 'the oncologist will talk to you about that...', 'they will decide if you should have surgery in a special meeting, the MDT...' 'You'll get an appointment very soon to see one of the lung doctors...'

Sometimes you *do* meet the patient again - if they become acutely unwell. This might be due to chemotherapy induced bone marrow suppression and sepsis, an inter-current pneumonia; anything that requires admission via the ED. They might just happen to be admitted when I am on call, just as they happened to come in under my care the first time. There may have been an interval of two months. She looks worse. You read the notes, and catch up on all that has been going on. Appointments here, procedures there, PET scans, problems… You wonder if any of the things you said came true. Did the oncologist discuss prognosis with you – did you ask him the 'big' question ('How long?') that you asked me? Did the appointment come through? Did you wait too long? Did the nurse specialist call you to keep you informed? So much has happened since that first shocked conversation by the bedside, curtains drawn, your husband leaning forward, staring at the tops of his shoes mutely…the day I broke the news and tapped into your deepest fears.

It is not possible to remain involved in every patient's journey, especially when their illness falls outside our own area of expertise. The best we can do, it seems, is deliver the first message skilfully and with conviction, while hoping that the promises we offer are realistic, and the undertakings we take on behalf of our colleagues are achievable. Beyond that, we cannot realistically hope to observe their progress or influence their experience. Trainees on the ward soon experience emotionally intense interactions that seem to be over just hours or days after they have begun. A working week might involve many such micro-relationships, and learning how to move nimbly - but not *too smoothly* - through this gauntlet of emotions is hugely important.

A little piece of you – care.data dialogue

This is my fanciful contribution to the care.data debate. For a more rational account please see Jonathon Tomlinson's recent blog post 'Care dot data', and Ben Goldacre's accounts in the Guardian. This article (A simple guide to Care.data by Olivia Solon) in Wired magazine is very readable too; it discusses Green, Amber and Red data, how much agencies will pay to get it, and the feasibility of re-identification.

My reading of the situation is that people are concerned about two aspects -

1) the possibility of their personal medical details ('secrets', a term used by Ben Goldacre) being accessed by strangers; an issue of confidentiality

2) the possibility that agencies who are not part NHS affiliated or research institutions with adequate governance structures will use it to increase profits; an issue of transparency

oOo

Two retirees, Geoff and Pat. They meet again to discuss care.data. Geoff has major reservations, while Pat continues to bang the drum. Pat has been doing a bit of work to bolster his argument, as Geoff will discover.

G   "Any more thoughts on this care.data controversy?"

P   "I still maintain, it sounds like a great idea."

G   "I'm opting out. No-one has got the right to see my medical details."

P   "But no-one wants to see *your* details. It's not personal."

G   "It is if the anonymisation code is broken. Or if someone cross-triangulates the information."

P   "But why would anyone want to do that? Why would they be so interested in your details?"

G   "Who knows. It's the principle, that it *can* be done."

P   "However unlikely that breach of confidentiality?"

G   "Yes, I worry that someone, at some point, might want to find out about my health."

P   "And you think that would be the best way to do it? Crack the care.data database. I'm sceptical."

G   "It's the lack of guarantee. There is no large, publically administered database that is immune to criminal interference."

P   "Well you can't substantiate that I'm sure, but many would agree with you. There is a trust issue that I'll come to. I'm just wondering though, whether to take a risk to make a point. You'll be very annoyed with me."

G   "Try me."

P   "You'll forgive me?"

G   "Let's hear it."

The open secrets

P   "OK. I wouldn't insure your life. I know that you have had rheumatoid arthritis since you were 35, that you need a new shoulder joint but are unlikely to get one, that your medication has recently been strengthened, that you require frequent monitoring of your immune system, and that two years you had a cancer scare that required you to stay in hospital for one week."

G   "Who told you?"

P   "No-one told me anything."

G   "Then how?"

P   "I was in the GP's last week. The blood samples were in a plastic basket near the front desk waiting to be picked up. Yours were at the top, and I read the form."

G   "Why on earth?"

P   "Well I wasn't going to shut my eyes was I. I looked in that direction, it was in front of me. And it said, *'RA 30 years, now on Aza.'* I know you are 65."

G   "And the rest?"

P   "I looked up Aza...it means Azathioprine. Powerful stuff, obviously only recently prescribed as it said 'now on'. And they're still monitoring you closely on it."

G   "Yes...and?"

P   "Two weeks ago I went to the hospital, to the out-patients clinic. You were there on the same day, and I was behind you in the queue to check in. The receptionist asked you who you were due to see, and you said Mr Chandler. I know he is an orthopaedic surgeon, and a shoulder specialist. Later I saw you leave - I was sitting in the coffee shop - and you were very down in the mouth. Hence my inference."

G   "Right little Sherlock aren't you. And the cancer scare?"

P   "Well, after your appointment you were sent for an MRI scan. I followed you to the radiology department."

G   "Why?"

P   "To hand in my own x-request actually, but also to prove my point. We had already spoken about care.data. So I stood in line again, and the receptionist there turned her monitor round to point out what availability there was. On the left of the screen, for anyone with half an interest to read it, was your history in that department. You've had countless joint x-rays, obviously, but one stood out, a PET scan. They are only really ordered if there is a concern about cancer. And the date on it coincided with the week you failed to turn up at the local history club a couple of years ago. Cancer scare."

G   "Christ on a bike."

P   "Sorry."

G   "You invaded my privacy."

P   "Privacy! You've been in hospital, you know what that word means - nothing! There is no privacy. If I had been in your ward I would have overheard every conversation that you had with your doctors, I would have heard their subdued, concerned tones as they broached the subject of possible cancer. I would have heard them explain the scan result, I would know everything. If you were ill and weak, I would have been aware of your every bowel

111

movement. In the hard end of healthcare, there is no privacy - just a pretence of privacy. You can be quite sure that much of your 'data', many of your medical details, were there to be seen when you stayed in hospital, but there was nobody to take note of it, because they had no interest in *you* as an individual. It's the same with care.data. It'll be there, protected quite well probably, but there will be nobody in a darkened room, the blinds pulled down, who wants to scrutinise your contribution to it."

Justified paranoia, or just squeamishness

G   "Your argument seems based on the assumption that naysayers like myself are either paranoid or have an over-inflated perception of their own importance."

P   "Paranoia, yes. Perhaps it's partly to do with the Snowden revelations, PRISM and all that. And there *is* an overlap. I discovered those things about you with barely an effort. Your data is out there already. Confidentiality is not about what people know, but what they do with the information. It's like the tree falling in the forest when no-one is there - does it still make a sound? Same with data. Your data could be seen, discussed, interpreted, all day every day for a decade, but it would only affect you, only enter your perception, if it led to a decision that touched you. It's just like the

NSA or GCHQ. I don't care if they read all my tedious facebook updates unless they come round and make something of it."

G   "That's naive. What if you were convening a new, subversive political party...would you feel quite so nonchalant then? Your medical details might become quite valuable. It would be very useful to know you needed insulin three times a day, should you start to cause trouble! It *is* naive to think that just because you and I are conventional, nefarious agencies will have no interest in picking out individuals' details and using them."

P   "But how many of us will ever be so significant as to attract that kind of attention? It's too fanciful! And I think the data to be uploaded is a little more cryptic than you might imagine. As I showed with my brief exercise in detection, anything that anyone wanted to find out about you they could discover much more easily by spending a couple of days in the neighbourhood. I have a more challenging proposition to put to you."

G   "Go on."

The philosophy of ownership

P   "...You don't own the data anyway."

G   "I do. It's my body."

113

P   "No. It's measurements that have been taken by a doctor, or conditions that have been diagnosed by them. The data wouldn't exist without them."

P   "It's still derived from me."

G   "*By* the doctor. And how did the doctor come to be there?"

P   "She's employed by the NHS."

G   "Yes, provided through the taxes that you pay."

P   "I don't see where you're going with this."

G   "The point I'm making is that your is the property of those who find it and compile it, in this case, the state, through the state health service."

P   "*I* am the property of the state?"

G   "Your data, yes. Just as the state owns your driving history, your legal history, they know which houses you've lived in, what grades you got at school - it's all data particular to you. What's different about your *medical* data?"

P   "It's *more* personal. It's from my body, it's about what's *in* my body."

G   "Are you sure it's not squeamishness, or the potential for embarrassment? Is it the possibility that someone can read about the episode of psychosis when you were 24, or the erectile dysfunction drug you were prescribed last year- I'm not talking about you, obviously - but in theory?"

P   "Perhaps it is. Medical details are different. They come into existence not because the state employs a doctor or a nurse, but because we choose to go and see those personnel, and trust them with our private concerns."

G   "So it's a matter of trust. That's the essence of it isn't it?"

P   "Yes. On several levels. The one-to-one trust that allows me to speak to my doctor..."

G   "You know, don't you, that hospital data is already uploaded. Each episode of care. The week you spent in hospital...that's in there somewhere. Anonymised. Diagnosis, outcome, your age, your comorbidities. You knew that?"

P   "I did. But this is different. It's longitudinal, it's my entire history in primary care. Much more personal. How can you argue that anyone but me can own it? It's *my* history."

G   "I suppose it goes back to Rousseau's Social Contract. It is the *general will* that we, the sovereign people, give our government the right and the privilege of choosing how to administer power in

115

our best interests. For our part, we have agreed to make sacrifices, in order to allow the general will to be advanced, such as resisting the temptation to take what we want - that is to behave anarchically, to give up part of our income - taxes, and, I would contend, to give up some of *ourselves*, in the form of information. Care.data is part of that sacrifice. We may experience a mite of discomfort, we may not enjoy the idea that a part of us resides in a database, but the general will, in this case to live longer, and to benefit from advances in understanding that might occur, outweighs that. The hitherto unrecognised patterns of disease, to be identified, or unanticipated associations between geography or employment or lifestyle and disease, may benefit future generations."

Those actuaries

P   "Yes, yes, I have accepted the advantages..but my misgivings remain, regarding transparency...motives. It is not the 'general will' that insurance companies refine their actuarial tables and maximize their profits…"

G   "Why not?"

P   "Why not! Why would I want them t make more money…from my data? And end up charging me more because I had a cancer scare!"

G   "But you are happy to be charged less for your car insurance than a 17 year old, based on the fact that you are a better prospect than the reckless youth. Is that different?"

P   "Yes."

G   "And you are happy to pay less for life insurance than a smoker?"

P   "Yes, but…"

G   "It is no different, in essence. They make that calculation because of data. Available data, about who lives and who dies. Cold, crude data that is comprised of numberless individual tragedies. But we need to know it."

P   "You seem to be an apologist for the state. You seem to have developed great faith in the wisdom of the state, although I seem to recall you opposed the Health and Social Care Act with equal sincerity. Not so wise all the time it seems. "

G   "I am vulnerable to the charge of naivety. But yes, I believe that care.data is a good decision, and that after this pause, when the furore has died down, we will reap huge benefits in the years that follow. It's just a shame they screwed it up so badly, for want of a sensible hand on the tiller, and an understanding of, and respect for, how people feel. Such a shame."

Two rooms

Doctors speak several dialects, and the contrast between that used with patients and that used with colleagues can be stark. I sometimes wonder how patients would react if they heard every conversation that concerned them?

Such a notion seems absurd, practically, though they surely have a right to such access. We have already been through a process of openness with letters, which used to be sent to GPs but not patients. There was a vogue to ask patients if they wanted to receive them, and now patients get them automatically (in my experience anyway). This has caused a change in the way letters are written, such that doctors tend to avoid opaque medical terms and provide more accessible explanations. Personally, I still write in a 'doctor- to doctor' way, as the GP is the primary recipient, but I know that if I use lots of acronyms or eponyms the patient will a) be excluded from the thought processes behind their management and b) likely to hold up a highlighted copy when I next see them in clinic.

But back to the conversations. If there is a suspicion of cancer, for instance, it is common to discuss a patient's condition and scan results in a multidisciplinary team (MDT) meeting. MDTs are designed to bring the opinions of several specialists to the table, for example: surgeons, oncologists, specialist physicians, nurses and dieticians. Some of these meetings go on for hours. Cases may require prolonged discussion, and can become heated if opinions are not in alignment. But other cases are easy, because it is clear that nothing to be done. The liver may be overwhelmed with infiltrates of cancer. Conclusion: no treatment options - palliative care only. Somebody might say, 'Hopeless'. They are not being heartless; they have never met the patient. But it's just true. Next patient. It may have taken no more than a minute to reach that conclusion. It is medicine at its coldest and at its most efficient. Time will be spent on the ones for whom there is a therapeutic option, a chance of cure or prolongation.

As soon as practically possible the patient is seen and the results are communicated to them. We move to the second room. As much time as necessary is taken to break the news, and, if done well, the scene will demonstrate medicine at its most compassionate. What a contrast.

If the patient had witnessed the MDT discussion they may well have been sickened by the speed with which their case was dismissed. What about all the other details? Their wishes, their social situation, their feelings... but no, those aspects were not relevant. It was, to be brutal, a technical decision. Too advanced for surgery; too frail for chemotherapy.

Each discussion has a distinct purpose, and each requires a different set of medical skills. To perform well in each environment a doctor has to adapt. Engage emotionally when required, but remain objective, scientifically accurate and evidenced based at other times. To bewail the lack of a more holistic discussion in the MDT would not be appropriate – it would not meaningfully contribute to the decision, and it would hold up the flow. The doctor or nurse in that meeting who actually knows the patient might find it *too* cold, and might experience a degree of dissonance as everything they have learnt about this unfortunate person is shorn from the presentation. But, come the face to face meeting, all those details come back into play, and are, of course, essential.

What does this contrast tell us? It suggests to me that there will always be a place for compartmentalisation. The modern, post-paternalistic culture, perhaps best summarised in the phrase 'no decision about me without me', seems to reach a limit in circumstances where highly focussed and specialised discussion must take place in a clear, unemotional atmosphere. MDT meetings are a necessary but, at times, somewhat surprising throwback to the sacerdotal, impenetrable practice of medicine in centuries past.

Interactive Ward Ethics 2: Dangerous

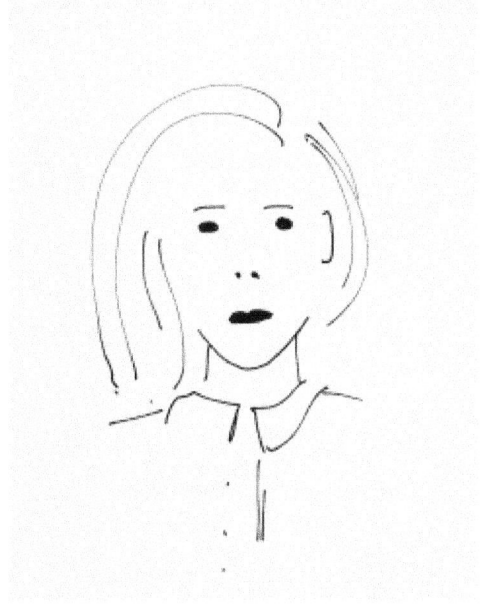

This is the second interactive post, and the scenario places our long suffering but excellent medical registrar, Nina Charan, in a no-win situation. She observes a colleague, another registrar, making a complete mess of a delicate medical procedure, and has to decide how to deal with it. Should she ignore it, manage it herself, give him time to improve, or escalate her concerns immediately? What may look obvious, from a patient safety point of view, becomes more challenging when you think about the psychology and emotional risks.

The choices you make for Nina will lead her into various stressful consequences, although some will result in a satisfactory outcome.

oOo

1.

Nina met the new registrar on the high dependency unit. She had heard good things about him, but as he had joined the hospital halfway through the year she had not had many opportunities to get to know him.

Nina had a complex patient whom she wished to discuss with him, but as she entered the ward she saw that he was in the middle of a procedure. He beckoned to her through a gap in the curtains, she entered, and he introduced himself with a friendly smile. Then he looked down and continued with this task, the insertion of a central line*. Nina described the details of her case in abstract, and David nodded. But Nina's attention was drawn to what he was doing to the patient. He seemed to be struggling to find the vein. The way he had organised his instruments and the way he held the ultrasound probe seemed strange. Her speech faltered and she found herself staring down at the pool of blood collecting around the patients shoulder, rather than concentrating on getting across the salient aspects of her own patient's presentation.

"Is this a hard one?" she asked.

"It is a bit, I just can't seem to…"

"How long have you been trying?"

"30 or 40 minutes. It's strange, everything seems to…"

Nina realised that she was being more of a hindrance than a help. As she left she ran into the patient's nurse, and she was shaking her head.

"Difficult one." commented Nina.

"Not really." replied nurse. The expression on her face indicated that at all was not well on the wall.

Later in the afternoon Nina found herself in conversation with one of the registrars that she knew well. Conversation moved on to the new registrar.

"What you know about it him?"

"Bit of a highflier I've heard. Ph.D., but he's from out of this region. I don't know him yet, no opinion." To this Nina this did not suggest a positive initial impression. Well, she would keep our eyes open. But…but…thinking about it, the technique David had been using for the central line was completely wrong. Did he actually know how to do it? Should she speak to somebody – escalate it? After just one observation? Did she have a duty to look into this in more detail? As she walked up the corridor, she considered her options.

Ignore it, go to 2

Have a word with David, go to 3

Escalate immediately to David's clinical supervisor, go to 4

* insertion of needle, then a wire, then a narrow tube for the delivery of drugs and fluids, into a major neck vein.

2.

The more she thought about it, the more it seemed inappropriate for her to act on this one observation. After all, David had arrived with a reputation. His specialty required expertise at vascular access. Nina had over-reacted. She resolved to focus on her own concerns.

Go to 8

3.

Nina passed him in a corridor. She paused, looked up, but said nothing and continued. Then she turned and caught up with him.

"Excuse me, David…" He stopped.

"Hi Nina…"

"I was just wondering…how did it go with that patient in the end, the one with the difficult central line?"

"Oh, I abandoned it, asked an anaesthetist to do it. Why?"

"It's just…oh, I felt for you actually, when they go wrong like that…"

"It was alright, it didn't go wrong as such, but I hit the carotid and it swelled up, I couldn't see the vein anymore…"

Nina changed tack. It was so hard to do this. "I trained before the ultrasound probes became routine. I was quite happy using landmarks, then I had to re-train. You?"

"No. I've used probes since I started."

"They can be a handful, can't they?"

David paused now. He was taller than Nina. "I've always got on pretty well with them."

"Sure, sure, I guess you use them all the time in cardiology, putting in pacing wires…"

"Yes, that's right. I do."

"Well, this Trust has a great simulator suite, and if you feel you're rusty, like I did after I came out of research, you can just go down there and book a session. It's really easy."

"Really. Is there? Look, I was *teaching* central lines in my last trust. I don't think I need any more training. But thanks for the advice, Nina. See you around." He left, evidently displeased.

Leave it, go to 8

Escalate to David's clinical supervisor, go to 4

4.

Nina knocked on Dr Stretton's door. She was David's clinical supervisor.

"Come in Nina, come in! How can I help you?"

"It's a bit difficult actually. It's about David, the new cardiology registrar."

"Oh yes. I haven't got to know him very well yet. Take a seat Nina, this sounds ominous."

"I watched him do a central line. He didn't have a clue."

"Right! OK. That's surprising. He's just come out of three years research in Newcastle, electrophysiology I think."

"That's what I thought. He must have been putting in lines every day."

"Was it a particularly difficult case?" asked Dr Stretton.

"I couldn't really say."

"Did you say anything to him?"

"No. Should I have?"

"No. I suppose not. Mmmm. So what do you think we should do?"

Nina was somewhat flummoxed. She hadn't thought of bringing a solution into the room. "What *can* we do?" she asked.

"The main question to ask ourselves is…is there a threat to patient safety? Sufficient to recommend that he be barred from doing central lines. Is there, from what you saw?"

"I can't really say that. From just one example."

"Well…what I do depends on what you saw, and how bad he was."

"Could you talk to him, ask him about his experience?" asked Nina, pushing back.

"I will, I will, don't worry. But I've seen his CV, his training is very comprehensive. I'll speak to him, but could you reflect on what you saw, and make a report. Get it down in writing or it never happened. Any particular circumstances, extenuating or otherwise. Then I'll decide what to do."

Find out more about circumstances, go to 6

Write report based on observations at time of central line attempt, go to 7

5.

Nina's bleep went off. She rang the number.

"Nina. Have you got a minute?"

It was Dr Stretton.

"I just wanted to say Nina...I made some enquiries about David. I'm so glad I did. And I'm so glad you came to me. His trainers, in Newcastle, had a lot to say about him. He's really had a lot of problems. The research was a bit of a distraction I think, from the main message. He's not going to be able to pursue an interventional career. He was probably deluding himself – I don't mind sharing it with you – and I'm thankful that we have found that out at *this* stage. Nina, what you did was very important. I know it wasn't easy for you."

Go to Summing up

6.

Nina described the situation, and what she knew of the patient. She felt that Dr Stretton was looking for some guidance herself, an impression on which to base her actions. So Nina had to grow up a bit, and form an opinion. She saved the file and walked around to the high dependency unit. Two nurses were preparing infusions in the clean room.

"Excuse me…"

"Hi Nina. What's up?"

"This new guy, David…what's he like?" The nurses exchanged glances. The first spoke, "Nice guy, really nice guy. Just had a baby, apparently. Keeping him up all night he told us."

"And clinically?" asked Nina.

"It's quite soon to tell," said the second.

"But…" pushed Nina.

"Perhaps he's a bit it out of practise. Research, you know…"

"How much out of practise? I'm not stirring, it's just important to support him, if anything…"

"Yeah, we know. That central line you saw was pretty bad. Not sure if he's got the hands, you know." Nina returned to her computer. – Do I recommend that he be re-trained? Really? What do I know…It's just one observation? He's sleep deprived…won't I be, when I have a child? What will it do to him, to be barred from a procedure that's so…cardiological? It's too early. But…but…would I want him putting a central line into my mother? No. No way. It's like he was wearing boxing gloves…

She wrote the conclusion:

A. 'I would recommend further observation of practise' >>>> go to 7

B. 'I would recommend a temporary restriction until his competence has been fully assessed' >>>> go to 11

7.

She wrote blandly. She resented this responsibility. Why had it come down to her words, her opinions? She wasn't senior enough. She wasn't in charge. She had witnessed one incident, that was all. She added something about the agitation of the patient, the sub-optimal conditions in which David had been performing. She tried to bring some balance. And she knew that based on this, Dr Stretton was unlikely to take strong action.

Go to 13

8.

Two days later Nina was on the night shift. At 9PM she entered the handover room and greeted members of the departing and arriving teams as they took their seats or perched on desks.

"What's Tracey up to?" she asked. Tracey had been on-call during the day.

"She's stuck on the ward, doing a chest drain I heard."

"Exciting! We don't get to do many of those anymore."

"It was an emergency. Somebody with a haemothorax*."

"How did they get that?"

"Failed subclavian central line insertion, and on some sort of blood-thinner, Clopidogrel I think." Nina felt cold.

"Where...where's the patient, what ward?"

"Cardiology." The handover was completed without Tracey. As soon as she was free, Nina rushed to the cardiology ward. Tracey was stitching the drain to the skin. She looked up and smiled, but her eyes were stressed.

"Disaster." she said.

"What...who...?" asked Nina.

"Guess." Nina opened the notes and saw David's handwriting. She resolved to get through the night, but at first light...she would do something.

Go to 21

* blood leaking into the space between lung and ribcage, a life threatening complication

9.

Nina couldn't let it end like that. She followed David up the corridor, and stopped him.

"No, sorry David, I can't just ignore what I saw. I've always found I best to be honest, I don't want to hide what I'm thinking. I really think you should go down to the sim suite and book a session. I can't make you…but we're all registrars together, we all have strengths and weaknesses, there are things you can do that I can't. But if anyone else sees to do a central line like that, there's a risk you'll be taken off the on-call rota…isn't there? But, as I say, I can't force you. But if there are any other mishaps, I'll have to speak to somebody. Sorry."

Go to 12

10.

She didn't want to escalate; it was the last thing in the world she wished to do. She was used to sorting out problems on her own…managing things without making a fuss. But speaking to David had achieved little. She walked to the consultants' offices.

Go to 4

11.

She had been dreading the moment. David was waiting in the line for a sandwich. Nina could not avoid speaking to him. But, there was no reason to think he knew it was Nina who had raised the alarm.

"How's it going?" she said.

"Me? Haven't you heard?"

"What?"

"They've taken me off the on-call rota."

"What?!"

"Completely. Because of central lines. Not trained! Someone must have complained, the anaesthetist probably…bit of an over-reaction, in my opinion."

"Oh. Yes. "

"I've been doing this for years! Years!"

"But…expectations are different now, you know, using ultrasound…"

"I can do it! It was just a difficult case or two! Just bad bloody luck!"

"Do they want you to do a bit of retraining?"

"Of course. But this has really messed up my chances…I was going to start a fellowship, that's the reason I came down from Newcastle. They won't have me now. No way."

"I'm sorry…"

"You?"

"For the…situation…I mean."

"Yes, right."

Nina left him. She may well have damaged his whole career – well, that was how it felt.

Go to 5

12.

"Keeping an eye eh, Nina?"

"Don't be like that David, please. How is it going? You OK?"

"If you're really interested…it's a difficult time actually. My baby has just come out of the paeds ward at St. Mike's, bad bronchiolitis…he was really poorly for three days."

"Was that…?"

"When you saw me mess up that central line? No, that was before, but it's been such a busy time. 4 hours sleep a night, tops. Do you have children?"

"No."

"Mmmm…it's tiring! I fall asleep on the bus every day. As soon as I sit down!"

"It must be difficult."

"It is. But…we carry on, don't we."

Nina felt as though she had been admonished, had her eyes opened to the 'real' world of childcare, where the demands of home had to be balanced with the demands of patients. Had she misjudged him?

Go to 17

13.

Three days later Nina was on the night shift. At 9PM she entered the handover room and greeted members of the departing and arriving teams as they took their seats or perched on desks.

"What's Tracey up to?" she asked. Tracey had been on-call during the day.

"She's stuck on the ward, doing a chest drain I heard."

"Exciting! We don't get to do many of those anymore."

"It was an emergency. Somebody with a haemothorax*."

"How did they get that?"

"Failed subclavian central line insertion, and on some sort of blood-thinner, Clopidogrel I think."

Nina felt cold. "Where…where's the patient, what ward?"

"Cardiology." The handover was completed without Tracey. As soon as she was free, Nina rushed to the cardiology ward. Tracey was stitching the drain to the skin. She looked up and smiled, but her eyes were stressed.

"Disaster." she said. "What…who…?" asked Nina.

"Guess."

Nina opened the notes and saw David's handwriting. She resolved to get through the night, but at first light…she would do something – or would she?

Go back to Dr Stretton, David's supervisor, go to 14

Discuss with David again, go to 15

Don't interfere, go to 16

* build up of blood in space between lung and ribcage, potentially lethal

14.

Nina hesitated outside Dr Stretton's door. This was déjà vu. Would she be interested? What more was there to say? Would it look as though she had some kind of personal problem with David? But no…she had to do it.

"Come in."

"Hi Dr Stretton."

"You look serious Nina."

"I need to tell you about another…incident."

"I think I've just had a phone call about it. Haemothorax patient?"

"Yes!"

"David?"

"Yes."

"OK. I'll have to take him off the medical rota. Don't worry, it's not just you."

Go to 11

15.

"Keeping an eye were you, eh Nina?"

"Don't be like that David, please. Are you OK?"

"I'm OK, unlike the patient…I hear."

Nina wanted to comfort him and explain it away for him; but she stopped herself. She tried to stay 'distant', while giving him the chance to talk about this.

"You look upset. Do you want to talk about it?" she asked.

"If you're really interested…it's just such a difficult time. My baby has just come out of the paeds ward at St. Mike's, bad bronchiolitis…he was really poorly for three days. And my wife was up in Newcastle on the day he got ill, where her folks are, it had to be the day she went away and asked someone to look after him. She feels awful about it."

"Was that…?"

"When you saw me mess up that central line on HDU? No, that was before, but it's been such a busy time. Four hours sleep a night, tops. Do you have children?"

"No."

"Mmmm…it's tiring! I fall asleep on the bus every day. As soon as I sit down!"

"It must be difficult."

"It is. But…we carry on, don't we?"

Nina felt as though she had been admonished, had her eyes opened to the 'real' world of childcare, where the demands of home had to be balanced with the demands of patients. Had she misjudged him? He was asking her to give him a chance.

Go to 18

16.

Nina had done her bit, she thought. The message had been passed, her concerns reported. What more could she do? So she waited, didn't watch too closely, and got on with her own life.

Go to 17

17.

It was something she had not planned. David just happened to be doing a procedure on a neighbouring ward. Nina asked a passing house officer what was going on. She was told that a patient with renal failure had come in, and the consultant had asked for a central line to be inserted on the morning ward round.

Nina walked tentatively onto the ward, and saw that the curtains had been pulled round the bed. David had a gown on, and was fumbling with the ultrasound probe. Nina nodded to him, and David did not ask her to leave. Nina could see the images on the ultrasound machine, and could see where the needle was approaching the large vessels in the neck. David's hand was pressing so hard on the neck that the vein was compressed and almost impossible to hit successfully. Not only that, both hands were shaking. Something, Nina knew what, had affected his confidence terribly. The wide bore needle in his right hand was pivoting in the skin. Nina could barely watch. The patient was awake, but had no idea what was going on through the blue haze of the sterile sheet that had been placed over her face.

Watch, go to 18

Ask David to stop, make him stop, go to 19

18.

Nina considered whether to take the ultimate sanction of asking David to stop, by physically removing him from the bed space. Such an action she would never have contemplated a few weeks ago. Contemplate she did – but no more than that. She watched, she justified her inaction.

With a hint from her, David released the pressure on the neck. The vein widened, and the needle approached. But still he was shaking. Nina hoped. It was too late to stop him now. The sharp tip of the needle must have been travelling a centimetre in either direction with each tremor. And then it entered the artery, and they could both see the tissue around it swell on the ultrasound screen.

"Oh." murmured David. "Oh."

"Just press. Pressure. Now!" urged Nina.

But he seemed to have frozen. He didn't do what he needed to do. Nina stepped forward, took some gauze squares, and pressed then down with her bare fingers on the swelling vessel. She called out, for a nurse. One appeared. David was just staring down.

"Can you please call Dr Stretton, and ask her to come? On her mobile if necessary. It's urgent. Just tell her it's very urgent."

Go to 23

19.

"David"

"What?"

"I don't think you should do this."

"What?"

"I don't think you should do this procedure."

"Nina, that's absurd. I've started. I'm almost there." "David, I really don't want you to continue."

"Come on, the patient… she's awake."

"Can talk outside for a minute? Please."

"No. We can't talk. This is important."

"David, please, I have something I need to tell you urgently." The patient had moved. The sterile sheet had slipped, and the situation had developed such that it was almost impossible for David to continue now. Reluctantly he set aside his equipment and followed Nina out into the main ward, his bloodied hands holding each other, almost in prayer, like an archetypal surgeon during an operation.

"I have to remove you from the situation David. I do not think you can safely perform this procedure. There, I've said it. It's come to this. I'm sorry I didn't do something earlier."

Go to 20

20.

Two days later –

"What a tale!" Dr Stretton spoke in the presence of Nina and the medical director. "He hasn't been trained properly at all. Some rather large assumptions made by medical staffing I'm afraid…"

"You saw his CV didn't you?" asked the medical director, pointedly, "Didn't you think it looked fishy?"

"I put my hands up. I saw he was five years into specialist training, I suppose I assumed he would have accumulated experience during his PhD. I was quite wrong. Thankfully, Dr Charan here did the right thing. Very brave really, many would have just turned away."

Thankfully, for Nina, she was not required to be present when they called in David.

Go to Summing Up

21.

But the night would not be so kind as to afford Nina the time to decide what action to take. Her initial prevarication would prove to have great consequences. As the sun rose she heard that the patient with the haemothorax had deteriorated further. She was on multiple organ support. After she had handed over the bleep in the morning she walked to the intensive care unit. She had to see what was going on.

Go to 22

22.

Nina entered the intensive care unit, and saw David standing calmly at the end of the bed, reading the notes. He looked up at Nina, then looked down again.

"What should I do?" she said to the side of his face.

"What do you mean?"

"About you."

"It's a recognised complication."

"I'm going to have to talk to someone. I wish I had already."

"Do what you want." He walked away. The intensive care consultant, Dr Bray, emerged from behind the curtain of a neighbouring patient. He had heard everything.

"What on earth is going on?" he asked, looking up the unit at the receding figure of David.

Nina told him everything.

oOo

The ICU consultant sat with Nina and Dr Stretton. Dr Stretton had heard it all too. Dr Bray said,

"She's probably going to die. She's got a severe lung injury, she's on maximal oxygen and her inotropes are rising. Kidneys are gone. This is very bad indeed, it's iatrogenic*. The indication to insert a central line was borderline anyway, but that's not the problem, it's the way it was done. And it seems that you, Nina, had reason to believe that David was not competent. Did you share this with anyone?"

"No. I thought…"

"It doesn't matter what you thought does it…it's too late."

"David was supposed to be fully competent, he's a senior trainee."

"Kath, what is his background? Do we know anything about him?" he asked Dr Stretton.

"More now I've made enquiries. His research was lab based. He went into it early in his training. He's only had a year as a specialist trainee, it transpires. We should have checked, we should have."

Nina felt the burden ease lightly. It was not all her fault. Dr Bray continued,

"Well, that will all come out at the Duty of Candour meeting, and perhaps the Coroner's. You'll be there…we all will."

Go to Summing Up

* Iatrogenic – 'relating to illness caused by medical examination or treatment'

23.

Nina took her hand off the gauze and stared down at the patient's neck; there was no further bleeding or swelling. She stood with David near the nurses' station. Dr Stretton entered the ward.

"What's the matter? What happened?"

"David was doing a…the introducer needle hit the carotid."

"Yes…so you press on it for 10 minutes. Was there something specific you needed?"

"I've let a…situation…get out of hand."

"What situation?"

"I observed David doing a central line a week ago, and I wasn't happy with his technique. I asked him about it, but he assured me he was competent. And today I saw that he was doing one and I came to watch, and it was the same story. Sorry, I should have let you know my concerns."

"Is the *patient* safe?"

"Yes, I think so. There's no more bleeding."

"Good, that's something. Come along, both of you. We need to talk this through."

Dr Stretton led, Nina followed, David came last.

Nina felt like a child in the playground, heading off to the headmistress's office.

Summing Up – Dangerous

What is the right course of action? The safest, to escalate concerns immediately, risks alienation, psychological stress, and the very simple risk that we are wrong about someone. The alternatives, that of waiting to see if there is a pattern of underperformance, or engaging the doctor privately, risks assuming too much responsibility. And who should we talk to? Can we be sure that the action they take will be reasonable or proportionate? If they overreact, will the underperforming trainee's confidence be irrevocably damaged, and the possibility of re-training them lost? These concerns are all focussed on what happens to the doctors involved, and not what happens to the *patients*. If there is a perceived threat to patient safety the answer comes more easily – act. That is our duty. But the grey areas, where there appear to be mitigating, and possibly self-limiting circumstances (a period of excessive fatigue for instance) – pose a very difficult challenge.

What would I have done here as a medical registrar, after the first incident? I really don't know. Probably, I would have spoken to David and explored his background in greater depth. Information gathering has to take place at some stage. But that means any further incidents over the next few days would be, partially, 'on me'. It's an unwinnable situation. That's why I wrote this, to illustrate the particular challenges that medicine, with its turnover of staff through institutions, their many and varied backgrounds, and the risk associated with the things we do, presents.

This Newsweek story tells, within a general discussion about hospital safety, how almost all members of a surgical audience put their hand up when asked if they knew a colleague who was 'dangerous'. Nicholas Shackel explores the morality of ignoring such colleagues in the Practical Ethics blog. The difficulties in tackling the problem are demonstrated in this piece about an underperforming pathologist, and finally, this link takes you to a helpful GMC page which touches on the subject of colleagues with medical problems or addiction related issues.

Candour crunch: being honest about risks on healthcare

The report *'Building a culture of candour - A review of the threshold for the duty of candour and of the incentives for care organisations to be candid'* makes very interesting reading. It seeks to define levels of harm that should trigger an approach to patients and relatives, and explores how organisations can be encouraged or compelled to develop a culture that facilitates this. It also touches on the realities of the 'post-paternalistic' era and the demonstration of candour in day to day practise.

Two excerpts:

'Modern medicine offers an abundance of hope, but very few absolute certainties. One of the comforts (some would say benefits) of paternalism was to obscure this lack of certainty for patients. This is no longer sustainable, and it means that being candid when things go wrong needs to be grounded in being honest about what could go wrong from the start. Better conversations about risk and the potential for harm are essential for fostering a culture of candour...'

'Clinical care is inherently risky, and while organisations and individual clinicians must do all they can to minimise those risks, it will never be possible to eliminate them fully.'

These appear to encourage a greater degree of upfront honesty about the risks of healthcare, rather than waiting for mistakes or unavoidable adverse events to happen before 'owning up'. We could, fancifully, call this 'pre-candour'.

I find the balance between upfront honesty and the provision of 'too much information' a hard one. Not all patients need or want the same depth of information about risk, even if, objectively, they face similar chances of accidental injury or death.

Opportunities to be open about risks begin in the Emergency Department or Admission Unit. Here I sometimes find myself explaining that coming into hospital is never routine, and that being on a ward brings with it physical and psychological risks. Sometimes this is part of the explanation as to why a patient should *not* be admitted. An example would be a young patient with a headache that does not sound suggestive of meningitis or haemorrhage; coming into hospital will not achieve anything, but they may have been led to expect admission to a ward, and may require convincing that it is right *not* to come in. The same might be true of a more elderly patient with a mild chest infection; they are weak and tired, they might benefit from three days in hospital, but if it is not entirely necessary, medically. A case may need to be made about why the

155

risks outweigh the advantages. One begins to speak of 'infections' or 'picking up bugs'. Is it appropriate to be negative about hospitals, and their inherent risks?

The 'hospitals are dangerous' mantra is unhelpful, but it is dishonest to portray hospitalisation in a neutral way. Henry Marsh, a (clearly disillusioned) neurosurgeon, wrote in the Independent newspaper recently that hospitals are

'... like prisons and there's a huge lack of insight into what a ghastly environment they are.'

This is depressing, but he has a point. An alert patient admitted to a general ward for more than a few days is likely to witness distress, disability, physical dependency, acute confusion, wandering, incontinence, the ravages of addiction and sadly, death at close quarters. Even with the most attentive and compassionate nursing, these aspects of frailty and illness cannot be hidden from the watchful. Patients of all ages have mentioned to me how eye-opening and challenging the experience of being an in-patient was. It does not seem unreasonable to explain some of these things in advance.

As to the physical dangers of hospitalisation, the degree of detail we should go into varies. Hospital acquired infections overall are less frequent nowadays (the incidence of MRSA and C Diff has fallen dramatically in recent years), but hospital acquired pneumonia does remain a common development in the frail population. Should we explain this, or quote the incidence? Do elderly patients and their families, who are coping with the news that they are ill and need to be admitted, need to be told that '...by the way, there's a chance you could catch something else as well...'?

A discussion about upfront candour is essentially a discussion about informed consent. In the context of planned procedures, this is clear and simple; we know which risks require explanation, the patient is enabled to understand these risks in relation to the benefits, and they agree or decline. But when we are discussing admission in the context of acute illness, the use of powerful antibiotics or drips that might facilitate the entrance of organisms into the blood stream, consent seems less relevant. The patient has no real choice about whether to come in or not. They are ill. To compound the stress of the situation by enumerating the additional risks may well be 'too much information'.

The post-paternalistic culture in which we work emphasises that patients are our equals, partners in care, and nothing should be hidden. However, we must surely remain sensitive to the fact that patients are also vulnerable, and may, in certain circumstances, be happy to 'have things done to them' without full and frank discussion. All doctors will recognise the scenario of the patient who has halted them mid-explanation with the phrase, 'Doc, just do what you need to do, OK.'

The key, it seems to me, is in modulating the degree of openness according to the patient's condition, its severity, its acuity, and the signals given off by the patient regarding their need for information. This modulation depends on the doctor's ability to understand the context and judge the person in front of them. Perhaps this requirement on the part of the doctor is *itself* paternalistic, as we are once again putting the *doctor's* interpretation centre stage.

Paternalism is always tempting. It makes life simple. As the authors of the report write, *'One of the comforts [ ] of paternalism was to obscure this lack of certainty...'* If things go to plan, and nothing goes wrong, the patient who was not been subjected to a conversation about risk will leave the hospital oblivious to the dangers that they faced, and their experience will in retrospect seem serene. If we are to encourage more 'pre-candour', we must be prepared to help our patients understand and accommodate the anxiety that may be engendered. This will require time to talk, time to listen, and time to answer. This is the price of candour, and of true partnership in healthcare.

Notes on a judgment

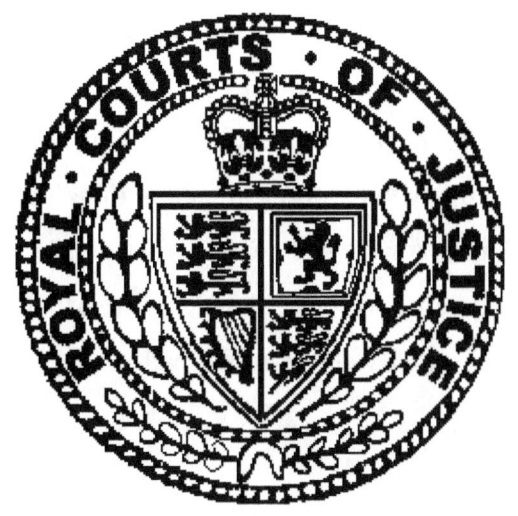

The judgment given in the case of Janet Tracey's estate vs. Cambridge University Hospital NHS Foundation Trust* contains lessons and warnings for doctors and nurses. There are fundamental implications, and there are subtle insights into how we go about discussing DNACPR decisions.

The judge wrote, in conclusion:

I would, therefore, grant a declaration against the Trust that it violated Mrs Tracey's article 8 right to respect for private life in failing to involve her in the process which led to the first notice [the first DNACPR form].

The following should be read on the understanding that i) I am not a human rights lawyer, and ii) I was not there, so the comments that I make on the communication that took place between doctors and patient/family are based only on what is written in the judgment. However, any messages or misunderstandings that I take away from the judgment as a physician with a general interest in resuscitation are likely to be repeated across the country. Also, the specifics of this case were in many ways atypical, and in thinking about what this judgment means for the rest of us, I have considered more common clinical scenarios – where patients are usually older, and perhaps on a more rapidly deteriorating path.

A mandatory discussion

The principle has now been established that not being given adequate opportunity to discuss your resuscitation status is an infringement on your 'right to privacy', that is, the right to lead your life how you choose without undue interference from the state. This is Article 8 of the European Convention on Human Rights. Thus the manner of dying becomes a subject of discussion that patients *must* be engaged in (unless it can be shown, clearly, that to do so would cause harm - see below). It sounds perfectly reasonable, and such engagement is already best practise. Respect for autonomy demands it, and few doctors complete DNACPR forms without trying their best to seek the patient's view.

But there are exceptions, and this judgment appears to belittle a doctor's right to use their discretion in extreme circumstances. It makes mandatory a discussion that in many cases is not relevant to the patient – that is, the option of trying to bring them back to life after they have died.

Patients with end stage disease admitted to hospital with a deterioration are often identified as entering the terminal phase. They will die naturally, and with good palliation they will die comfortably and with dignity. Cardiopulmonary resuscitation (CPR) has no place in this paradigm of care. It is never going to be effective, helpful or kind. But CPR *is* there, it is 'available', and the judgment seems to have made it illegal not to discuss its merits with all such patients (and/or relatives in the case of mental incapacity).

My assertion that CPR is often an *irrelevant* option may sound paternalistic. This requires examination, because there appears to be a discrepancy between how important doctors feel CPR is, and how important patients or families feel CPR is.

The diminishment of a symbol

Experienced hospital doctors will have seen scores of patients fail to recover from CPR, and will have witnessed many CPR attempts that are cut short after a minute or two once the insanity of the situation becomes clear. To many doctors CPR has become an unwelcome and frequently harmful intrusion on the natural deaths of frail or end-stage patients who receive it 'by default' - because their teams did not discuss it openly before the cardiac arrest occurred. All patients who die in hospital *will* be subjected to CPR unless a DNACPR decision has been made first. Thus the accumulation of many such regrettable experiences leads to an overall impression that CPR is over-used. Its apparently transformative potential – to bring people back to life - is diminished.

However, for patients and families CPR means something else. It is the very last hope of salvage when the patient's medical condition has deteriorated. It can be symbolic of a person's 'will to live' or their 'fight for life'. It cannot be dismissed as an irrelevance, even if it will surely not work. This, I think, is what the judgment reveals and concretizes into legal precedent – CPR, for all its fallibility, is too important to patients and families not to be made aware of its existence and its withholding.

Most in the medical profession know this already and accept it, but my concern is that in those circumstances when it is truly inappropriate there will be anxiety on the part of the doctors that DNACPR has not yet been discussed with the patient or the family. I worry that in such cases CPR will be given to avoid the accusation, after the event, that the patient's human rights were overlooked. The doctor's instinct, and all their experience in such situations, may be overridden by a defensive mindset.

I will now look at some specific lessons contained in the judgment.

Documentation of the discussion

Janet Tracey did not want to talk about her end of life care, according to the doctor who wrote the first DNACPR order. He is quoted as saying,

"Mrs Tracey did not wish to engage in discussion relating to her care and prognosis. On occasions when I attempted to initiate discussions with Mrs Tracey regarding her treatment and her future she did not want to discuss these issues with me."

This impression is backed up by the patient's husband who indicated that,

'Mrs Tracey felt "badgered" by the attempts of the doctors to discuss her end of life treatment with her.'

Ultimately however, the doctor did achieve some sort of interaction with the patient. In the judge's words,

'It was Dr _____'s evidence that he broached the issue of DNACPR with Mrs Tracey, explained what it meant and that she nodded to indicate her agreement to it. He then completed the *first notice*.'

She nodded. This was sufficient, in the eyes of the doctor, to be taken as agreement. However, the judge is concerned that,

'If Dr _____ had such a conversation, it would have been of importance to note the same both on the DNACPR Notice and in the medical records. I am unable to accept that the absence of such a note is a result of no more than poor record keeping.'

and,

'There is nothing in the medical/nursing records which suggests any agreement to DNACPR by Mrs Tracey. The tenor of entries prior to 4 March 2011 indicate that Mrs Tracey either did not agree or requested that any such discussion take place in the presence of her husband or daughters.'

thus,

'In the absence of any documentation and in the light of what is known about Mrs Tracey's view on the issue of resuscitation around the time of the first Notice, I am *unable to accept Dr _____'s evidence* that he spoke to Mrs Tracey about resuscitation prior to the implementation of the first DNACPR Notice.'

The judge does not believe that a DNACPR discussion took place. There was nothing to back it up.

Distress vs. harm

The average doctor's defence for not discussing DNACPR in a situation where it is plainly inappropriate to resuscitate, is that it would be positively unkind to bring it up with the dying patient. To steer the conversation towards a procedure after death that cannot work seems perverse…and may cause distress. This case hinged around the issue of distress, or a doctor's fear that to discuss DNACPR explicitly would cause distress.

We have seen how Janet Tracey appeared unwilling to engage in discussions about death. It is reasonable, in my opinion, to assume that forcing her to talk about it would have caused distressed. In light of the concern that to insist on a discussion would be unkind, the judge accepts that,

'It may well be that such a concern also caused him to spare her a conversation which he knew was likely to cause *distress* to a suffering patient.'

But the judge does not feel that 'distress' is sufficient reason *not* to insist on that discussion. Hence,

'In my view, doctors should be *wary of being too ready to exclude patients* from the process on the grounds that their involvement is likely to distress them.'

and,

'Many patients may find it distressing to discuss the question whether CPR should be withheld from them in the event of a cardio-respiratory arrest. If however the clinician forms the view that the patient will not suffer harm if she is consulted, the fact that she may find the topic *distressing* is unlikely to make it inappropriate to involve her.'

Only if we feel that the discussion will truly cause harm does there appear to be an exemption;

'There can be little doubt that it is inappropriate (and therefore not a requirement of Article 8 to involve the patient in the process if the clinician considers that to do so is likely to cause her to suffer physical or psychological harm.'

In these cases we will need to be very clear, in the notes, as to our reasoning that harm may occur. I am not sure how we as doctors will articulate that reasoning. When does distress become harm? Isn't any distress harmful, in the context of the dying phase? Or should we accept that dying is distressing anyway, and a little extra distress is a small price to pay for obtaining our patients' full opinion on the matter? We need to come up with an answer to this.

Clarity, brutality

It seems that the doctor failed to be clear with the patient's family member about what DNACPR actually was. After having a discussion about it with a doctor she left the hospital, but then looked up what the decision meant in more detail, on the internet. Having realised that her mother actually being deprived of a potentially life-saving intervention she came back to the team with a challenge, and the order was rescinded.

The judge writes,

'…whether in a wish to spare her the harshness of a graphic explanation of CPR or a belief that in using words such as 'slip away' he was conveying the entirety of such a scenario, I believe that the entirety of the position was *not fully understood by* _____"

167

This rings true. It is very easy not to go into great detail, and there are several reasons for this. Primarily, I believe, doctors who have already made the medical decision that CPR is not appropriate are unwilling to describe its ins and outs because to do so is, once again, irrelevant. It distracts from the subject of most importance, how to manage symptoms *in life*, not what to do *after death*. If 'graphic' descriptions are given, it can begin to feel positively gratuitous. However, one lesson that this judgment provides is that we should make very sure that the relatives of our patients do understand. That may require some unpleasant conversations, and not a little emotional harm. We must learn how to do this well.

An allowance

The judge seems to make some provision for difficult cases. It should be remembered that the focus of this case was a mentally capacitous patient's apparent unwillingness to be involved in discussions, and the doctors perception that to engage her in the discussion would be psychologically harmful – the judge was not convinced about this, and did not find written evidence in the notes to support the doctor's case. The judge writes,

'I recognise that these are difficult issues which require clinicians to make sensitive decisions sometimes in very stressful circumstances. I would add that the court should be *very slow to find that such decisions, if conscientiously taken, violate a patient's rights* under article 8 of the Convention.'

The obverse

Finally, this judgment can be read the other way round. Having established that talking about one's treatment after cardiac arrest is important enough to require legal protection, we must consider the situation where CPR is performed when the patient *would not have wanted it*. The legal principle of anticipatory discussion applies both ways, as highlighted in a Resuscitation Council statement released shortly after the judgment. Basically, it is as irresponsible to permit, through failure to discuss, inappropriate CPR as it is to withhold it. They write,

'*The RC (UK) considers that Article 8 may be engaged and potentially breached also should a clinician* **not consider an anticipatory decision about CPR with or for a patient who is at clear risk of dying or suffering cardio respiratory arrest**. *Failure to consider a decision about CPR or to ascertain the patient's wishes in relation to CPR (or the views of those close to the patient without capacity) may leave such a person at risk of receiving CPR that they would not have wished to have and that could have been avoided had the matter been afforded appropriate consideration and discussion.'*

The message is - think about CPR early, talk about it bravely but sensitively, and write everything down.

oOo

* A case was also brought against the Secretary State for Health, in relation to his possible duty to ensure a standardised DNACPR policy for the NHS. I will not go into that part of the judgment here, although in summary, the appeal court found that there was no obligation on him to impose a centrally designed policy.

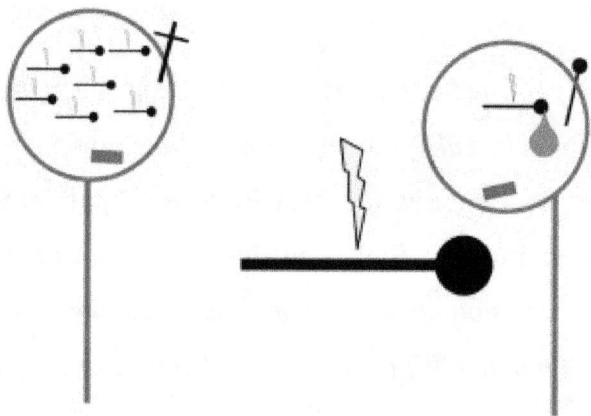

The turning away

When I tell him that his liver is so badly diseased it may not recover, he turns away and looks into the middle distance. There are no questions. He was expecting this. He has probably known that it would end like this for several years, perhaps a decade. But even this foreknowledge could not change his behaviour. He continued to drink, and now, at the age of 4_, he is approaching the end of his life.

I want to ask him why he couldn't stop. Naïve I know – but doesn't the prospect of death outweigh the immediacy of compulsion? After all, he was well supported at home; he had every opportunity to arrest the damage in its tracks and live to a decent age. I would like to know why…what was going on in there? But we are well past that now. Serious complications have set in, and all I can do is treat each one as it develops. He clearly doesn't want to talk about it, and I am not comfortable pushing him.

When all the patient really needs is treatment there seems to be little place for such enquiries. The answers will add nothing; the questions will do no more than suggest to the patient that *he did this…he had a choice*. In contrast to patients who hold our gaze with a combination of anxiety and confusion, and ask 'Why me?', the alcoholic has all the information he needs. Whatever the truth, wherever the blame lies, those factors are irrelevant now. That's why he looks away. There is nothing to say, nothing to explore.

Understanding why patients made certain choices does not allow us to reach into the past and shake them to their senses, or reveal to them a picture of their future selves – debilitated, jaundiced, desperate. A fortunate percentage will survive their first emergency, and with abstinence will see their liver improve. Some may even be judged appropriate to receive a new liver. But what of those who continue to deteriorate, and who in turning away seem determined to keep their personal truth to themselves? Does this aversion to allowing us beneath the surface impair the quality of care that is given?

It might. Doctors are not brilliant at digging into patients' private lives or hidden histories. If, through an embarrassment of regret, a patient seems unwilling to discuss the behaviour that resulted in this crisis, the path of least resistance may lead doctors to a superficial degree of emotional engagement. Deeper knowledge of the patient is not acquired, the picture remains sketchy, and empathy does not develop. This may translate to a failure of advocacy. Doctors, who spend their days trying to determine if and when to escalate or intensify care, need to know that the patient *wants* to recover. They are driven, in large part, by the patient's expressed wishes. If the patient appears determined to survive, and says as much - 'I don't want to die doctor, please do your best to get me through this, I want to deal with this…' - the medical team is more likely to advocate for intensive care or prolonged support. Patients who remain silent and closed may appear uninterested in their own survival.

I worry that those who turn away deprive themselves of the opportunity to be known or understood, and are subsequently less likely to receive the best that medicine has to offer. The challenge, for those of us who receive them on the ward, is to prise away the (un)emotional armour and find out what they are really thinking. It's not comfortable, it may feel intrusive, but it is probably necessary.

Patterns and pride: diary of medical anecdote

...There is, it seems to us,

At best, only a limited value

In the knowledge derived from experience.

The knowledge imposes a pattern, and falsifies,

For the pattern is new in every moment

And every moment is a new and shocking

Valuation of all we have been.

T.S. Eliot, East Coker (Four Quartets)

Day 1

It was a good day today. There are not many occasions when you recognise the clues, feel bold enough to make a diagnosis, and see admiration in the eyes of your colleagues – some of whom didn't even know who you were.

The patient came in with fever, he was referred as just another pneumonia or a urinary infection, but I noticed that one of his blood results was unusually high. The eosinophils. This led me to ask about his travel history, because these cells often go up when there are parasites in the system. And indeed he had travelled, a fact that no one else had thought to ask. I looked up the country in which he had spent time, and worked out what sort of parasites could be involved. But I knew which one already. The symptoms seemed to fit what he was describing, to the letter. Fever, abdominal pain, some weight loss, and especially breathing difficulties that he had developed just before coming to hospital. It all fit.

So I looked up the treatment, called the pharmacist to make sure we had it in stock, and prescribed it. By the end of the day he was already feeling better. It made all the study seem worthwhile. But it was a special memory that served me so well today. I had seen a patient just like this one during my elective, in Africa. I even wrote about it in the report that we had to hand in, so it stuck in my brain. *Strongyloides*. I suppose, over a whole career, many such images and stories will find a place in my memory, to be retrieved at a later date. Nothing wasted, they all find a niche. A good day.

Day 2

I went straight into see him as soon as I arrived. He was grateful, and asked how long it would take him to get better. I said I would refer him to the tropical disease specialist, as they see more of this sort of thing. And of course I explained that we needed to confirm the diagnosis, even though I was pretty sure about it. I reviewed his blood tests, and saw this kidneys weren't working so well. He must have got very dehydrated before he came in. His breathing had settled slightly, but he was still struggling. I didn't want to come across as an expert, because I have only ever seen one other person with this. But he's on the right track.

Day 3

I was disappointed today. His kidneys were worse, despite the fluids that I prescribed. My consultant didn't have any new ideas, she was pretty happy to go along with my explanation. But she was keen to see confirmation of the diagnosis. The antibody tests will take days, they have to be done in London. She asked me whether it could be any other parasite, or any other type of infection full stop. Perhaps she doesn't quite trust my impression. It made me think, and reflect. But I've seen the list of parasites, and none of the others that he might have acquired in Africa present like this. So I suggested that we push on with the current treatment. It worked last time, I explained.

Day 4

Weird. He was confused today. This parasite can affect the brain though. I spent 45 minutes on the phone trying to get through to a tropical disease expert, to see what they thought. They agreed, yes, Strongyloides *can* go into the brain. So I arranged a scan, and it's happening after hours tonight. The anti-parasitic agent we're giving him will kick in soon.

Day 5

I went to see him but he wasn't there. I ran into another SHO in the corridor who had been on call overnight and he told me he'd been transferred to the intensive care unit. I almost ran. When I got there I found him unconscious, on a ventilator. He was surrounded by other doctors. There was a neurologist, examining his eyes. I asked what was going on. He had blown a pupil, I was told. It didn't make sense. I saw a nurse returning from one of the computers. She was shaking your head. 'What!' shouted one of the other consultants, a rheumatologist. *'They must have done it!'* he said. I faded into the background, but I continued to listen. What angered him was the fact that during the patient's entire admission, no one had sent off a vasculitis screen. As soon as I heard that word, vasculitis, my heart dropped and the muscles in my legs grew week. I had to sit down behind the nurses' station. I realised that I had made a huge mistake. For vasculitis is another main reason for eosinophils to be raised. I knew immediately what is the diagnosis was. Churg-Strauss syndrome. I had missed it completely.

Day 9

I met with my clinical supervisor today. I had asked for the meeting. I told her what happened. I could tell that she thought my mistake was a bit stupid. She asked me what my thought processes were on the day the patient came in. I explained the whole story, how it rung bells in my mind, how the words that he used, and the clinical examination findings, had taken me back to a vivid moment in my training. And I *had* questioned the data, and I *had* tested the hypothesis, and it all seemed to fit.

'But what about the differential diagnosis?' she asked

'I... I...'

'Did you develop one?'

'I did, I think. I'm n...'

'Did you write it down Emma, in the clerking? Did you test for anything else?'

'I didn't think I needed to. It was so clear.'

'Well, to be fair, the patient saw a lot of other people, and more senior than you, before he got really ill. No one really challenged the diagnosis. There's a lesson for all of us. But it shows you the power of a positive diagnosis. Especially one that appears to be supported with confidence. You're a junior doctor, but you see how much weight people give the opinion of anybody who seems sure of themselves. Yes, diagnoses should be challenged by more senior doctors as they review patients, but it is not uncommon for them to defer to the opinion of the first doctor who really got their teeth into the case. And that was *you*. You made a plan, it made sense, the patient even got a little bit better at first. Sometimes, I think, there is really one chance to set things into motion in the right direction, and that's on the first day of admission. It's a big responsibility. Am I making you feel any better?' She smiled. Then she asked, 'What would you do differently next time?'

'I won't be so confident.'

'That would be a shame, if you are right.'

'Well if I really think I'm right, I will make my case confidently. But I will make sure there are caveats, and that other avenues aren't closed off right at the beginning. Perhaps in this case, because he had raised eosinophils, he should've seen a rheumatologist anyway, even if I really thought he had an infection.'

179

'I'll tell you what I take away from this. The power of anecdote. In your mind there was a clear story, and narrative that you had seen played out before, one with a happy ending. You were sucked back into that memory. If you're like me, your memory works best when it's embedded in stories. But I guess that might be a disadvantage, if you can't stand back and approached each case with pure objectivity. Attack each case with fresh eyes, but use the stories that you recollect to remind you of all the possibilities.'

'I hear you.'

'And one more thing. The Procrustean Bed."

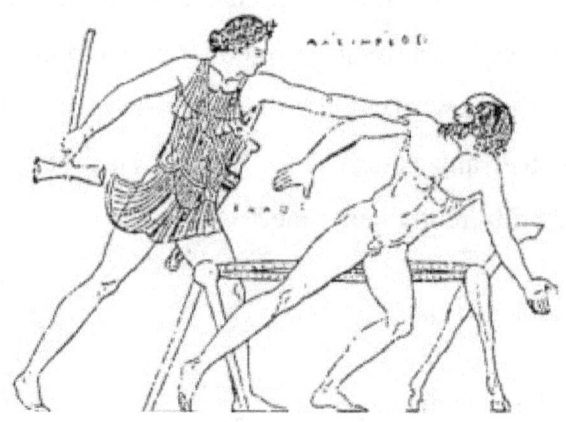

'The what?'

'His confusion. It challenged your hypothesis, it didn't make sense, but you rationalised it, and made it fit your idea – a parasite in the brain. Procrustes chopped or stretched travellers who encountered him until they fit the size of his bed. You not only fell into the trap of anecdotal memory, but you tailored your interpretation of the data so as to support it…'

'There is *one* more thing.'

'Tell me.'

'I was *pleased* with myself, on the first day. I elated, to make a difficult diagnosis.'

'That may be the most valuable lesson of all. It's seductive, the warmth that being right gives you. But don't worry, you'll experience enough reverses in your career to learn that pride is never to be entertained. I think you've learnt enough from this particular case, don't you! How is he by the way?'

'Getting there.'

- - -

Note: This case report from the CLEVELAND CLINIC JOURNAL OF MEDICINE explores the clinical scenario in more detail.

A gift freely given: dialogue on organ donation

This week it was announced that liver transplants would be offered to 'heavy drinkers' in a pilot programme. Patients will be young (typically less than 40) and will have such severe liver disease that the chance of them surviving the hitherto accepted period of 4-6 months of abstinence are remote. This has raised concerns that people will be less likely to sign up to be organ donors.

Here two people discuss donation. A has been put off by the idea that active drinkers might receive his liver, while B takes a more philosophical stance, and challenges A's hesitancy.

After the main dialogue there are extended footnotes on changes that have been made to organ donation law in Wales ('soft opt-out') and on the involvement of families in the decision to allow organ to be retrieved.

oOo

A "I was keen to donate my organs when I died, but I'm not so sure now. They're going to give livers to drinkers now, without even making sure that they can stop. It's crazy. I know they can't help it, I know there are a million back stories and life events that lead to alcoholism, but I think it gives the wrong message – don't worry too much, if your liver packs in there's a chance you could be rescued. Well I'm not sure I want to be one of those who gives a liver only for it to be ruined within a year or two by their addiction. We do all have the ability, and the strength, within us, to stop drinking…if we want to."

B "So it's weakness. They should be allowed to die because they are weak?"

A "They have a death wish, that's what I'm saying. Whatever the reason for them not being able to stop, and perhaps it doesn't really matter, the fact is that if they are given a new liver what's to say they won't carry on drinking."

B "But you realise, don't you, that you can have no idea who will get your liver. It could go to a teenager who stupidly overdosed on Paracetamol, a haemophiliac who contracted hepatitis C from contaminated blood products, or a blameless sufferer of inherited disease. Or half of it could go to very young child. If you don't give your liver, then it will be harder for those people to be treated. You can't predict or determine who gets it."

A "But the chances of it going to an alcoholic will be higher. And as I say, I don't like the message it gives. There's so much…latitude nowadays. For patients who have inflicted damage on themselves."

B "So is it a political or social comment that you will make by not donating? An attempt to influence society in some way."

A "I wouldn't say that."

B "But it's your opinion on the subject of addiction that is being translated into your decision not to donate."

A "Well…it is my decision, after all. It's my body."

B "You presume it is, but you will be dead."

A "Are you suggesting the state takes ownership?"

B "Legal ownership is a vexed question, but the more relevant question is how the state manages your right to decide."

A "Involuntary inclusion on the register of donors has been considered and thrown out, hasn't it. The 'opt out' was debated in Wales, I don't know what came of that [1]. But what you're suggesting is 'no opt out'! That's extreme. That sounds like the Chinese prisoners [2]."

B "Imagine this. Imagine another person, a hundred miles from here, having the same conversation with a friend. And imagine he is intending to put himself on the register of donors but is equally uneasy about, say…a convicted criminal receiving his liver or kidney or whatever. He wants to add a caveat to his donor card, that his organs can go to anyone as long as they have not been convicted of a serious crime in the past. What do you think of that?"

A "I recognise the intention, and sympathise with it, but I also recognise that it's probably not practicable. Better to just not donate if there are going to be stipulations or exclusions. Because, as you say, you can't control who gets your organs."

B "So this man will not donate. Another lost donor. And taking the argument further, there may be people who are uneasy about other groups receiving organs, ethnic groups, religious groups, or those with different sexual orientations. They too will have no choice but to not donate. In fact, if we accept that anyone with any concerns about their organs being used to prolong the life of another about whom they have some moral or religious or racial misgiving should probably not go on the register, then we have automatically shrunk the pool of organs by a considerable percentage. Having made a great advances in the science of transplantation, we now elevate the instinctive judgements, dare I say prejudices, of people above the opportunities that their organs might provide. Does that sound right?"

A "But hang on. You've gone from alcoholics to minority groups in one leap. None of those groups will be engaged in anything specific to their identity that will damage the liver. I'm not refusing to donate because I don't want some other person to survive – what do you think I am! - but because I don't want my liver to be wasted."

185

B "That's been considered. The trials show that the rate of liver wastage is no higher than in other groups, because the alcoholism is monitored and treated intensively. You know about Hepatitis C? Well, that always recurs in the new liver if it is not eradicated before the transplant (which it rarely is), and very large numbers of donated livers are used to replace previous transplants that have been re-infected. So many of the livers being given now are what you might call 'wasted', except they were not wasted because the patients benefitted hugely from receiving them. The 'waste' argument is a weak one. What I want to pin down is this - do donors have any right, any right at all, to have a view on the moral or character background of potential recipients?"

A "As normal, opinion-forming human beings, we are all bound to have a view. If I donated a liver and somehow knew, in the afterlife, or more to the point if my family knew, that it had gone to a previously convicted, albeit rehabilitated et cetera et cetera child-killer, I would be so angry."

B "Your family would be angry. You'd be dead."

A "Yes, my family would be angry. And they have a right to an opinion too."

B "OK, so you wish to transfer your objections to your family after death."

A "They are the natural inheritors of a potential donors wishes and concerns, aren't they?"

B "It's arguable."

A "Are you now suggesting that families have no say in this?"

B "They will bring their own moral structures and pre-judgments into the argument."

A "No, they will do their best to express what they think I felt about it. They are the best placed to do that."

B "And you think families can do that without colouring the subject with their own opinions?"

A "I don't know. But they have to be consulted."

B "You're right, families can veto organ donation, even if the patient made it clear that he or she wanted to donate. Doctors won't take organs in the face of strong opposition, and whether that it acceptable or not has been debated at length [3]. But let's assume your decision, taken before death, is carried through. How do you reconcile your understandable concerns about who might get your organs? This is how I feel about it. If you would receive an organ from a random person, then you should agree to donate to a random person. And if you do decide to donate, as an act of altruism to humanity, then you should accept that the range of possible recipients will include all that humanity has to offer. All sorts. And you should trust that the donation system will have in place checks to reduce as much as possible the risk of 'wastage', be it through drinking, or recurrent hepatitis C, or repeated overdoses...the essential decision is Am I happy to help my fellow man or woman who will die without a transplant? Am I happy to make that contribution to society, even despite the fact that there are some aspects of society that I do not like, and do not sympathise with. Have I persuaded you?"

A "Your reasoning has. But what you miss, I think, is that the decision is an emotional one. That's the trouble you see. People are led by their hearts, not their minds."

Footnotes

1] China

Executed prisoners have their organs harvested (without prior permission), although it is said that this practise will soon come to an end.

2] Wales

A 'soft opt-out' has now been passed into law and will come into effect in December 2015. This means that people living and dying in

Wales will be assumed to have given their consent unless they have made the effort to opt-out. This checklist is from the Organ Donation Wales website.

You will be treated as though you want to be an organ donor unless:

- you have already registered a decision to be a donor (opted in) or
- you have already stated you do not want to be a donor (opted out) or
- you have appointed a representative to make a decision about consent on your behalf or
- you lack capacity to understand that your consent could be deemed or
- a person in a relationship to you objects at the time of your death, on the basis that they knew you did not want to be a donor

In 2008 the Organ Donation Taskforce looked into what effects an opt-out system might have attitudes to donation. It took a very cautious view. It referred to experiences in Brazil and France:

There are two examples of a negative impact of presumed consent policies. Brazil adopted a 'hard' presumed consent law in 1997, with opt out denoted by a note on an id card or driving licence. The law had to be repealed in 1998, principally because of mistrust of government and accusations of body snatching.

In France, which has a variation of presumed consent, there was an incident in 1992 in which corneas were taken from a 19-year-old road traffic accident victim whose parents had consented to only limited organ retrieval. This resulted in a great deal of negative press coverage of the medical profession, despite the clinicians having complied with the strict letter of the law, and damaged public trust in the organ donation system for some time.

They concluded that....

[we are] not confident that the introduction of opt out legislation would increase organ donor numbers, and there is evidence that donor numbers may go down.

3] *The family veto*

The role of families hit the headlines in 2012, when David Shaw (a lecturer in medical ethics) wrote an article in the BMJ criticising the medical profession for acquiescing to the family veto, especially when the deceased had put their name down on the donor register. In an interview he stated that 1 in 10 families acted in this way, and a higher proportion refused donation when asked about donation and the patient was not on the register. He suggested that families often regret this decision because they have denied their relatives express wish, and also the fact that 'their decision may have caused deaths or suffering for other patients.'

The Organ Donation Taskforce also examined the role of families. It felt that their opinion was important, and that the decision to donate should rest in their hands.

There is an argument, advanced by some, that a system of presumed consent would relieve families of the burden of making a decision in the absence of any indication as to the deceased's wishes. The Taskforce finds this a somewhat paternalistic view, at odds with the ethos of today's NHS. Further, our evidence from donor families was that they stressed the importance to them of being involved in the decision to donate and of being allowed to make the decision that was right for them at the time. The Taskforce found the evidence from donor families compelling.

Additionally, the taskforce also found that recipients preferred to know that the donated organ had been given 'freely' and that the family was in agreement.

Recipients of transplants reported that it was important for them to know that the family of the donor had been involved in the decision and were comfortable with it. They also stressed the importance of knowing that organs had been freely given. These families spoke movingly of the concept of organ donation as a gift, and were concerned that an opt out system might undermine the principles of organ donation as a gift.

They concluded that systems where the opinion of families was not taken into consideration

...has the potential to erode the trust between clinicians and families at a distressing time. The concept of a gift freely given is an important one to both donor families and transplant recipients. The Taskforce feels that an opt out system of consent has the potential to undermine this concept.

The Christian Medical Foundation Head of public Policy, Phillipa Taylor, expressed her concerns about the exclusion of the family in this decision in a September 2012 blog post. With regard to ownership of the body in the context of an opt out system, she wrote,

The assumption about whose body it is begins to move from personal ownership to state ownership. Unless the state wishes to suggest that the deceased now belongs to it, the family must have the right to become his/her spokesperson.

As we have always said, CMF is supportive of organ donation in principle. However we are not supportive of presuming consent when it has not been given, nor do we support overriding the family and the important role they should play. God designed human beings in His image to be relational (Gen 1:26,27, 2:18-25) and the Bible everywhere assumes the significance of the family.

It seems the 'soft opt-out' system adopted in Wales has taken these views into consideration.

Leadership – the immediacy of example

Leadership, I am sure, takes many forms, but explicit exposure to the theories and approaches that might have helped develop doctors of my generation was lacking. The leadership that I was conscious of, as a trainee, was the example set by my seniors. Thus, as a consultant myself, the most direct route to leadership that I have identified is the example *I* give. This may be one-dimensional, and I hope that over the years other ways will reveal themselves.

The trouble with leading by example is that we are, as fallible people, inconsistent. In medicine inconsistency is risky. After several years on the wards it is possible to recognise how the example one sets can translate, directly, into the care that is delivered. In this post I try to relate how that translation can occur with a short account. It is not a sophisticated scenario, but one that shows how healthcare, more than other profession perhaps, can excel or fail due to the behaviour and attitudes of those in charge.

oOo

A busy ward round - Monday. The consultant, Dr Blackburn, paces himself. He intends to see all the patients, but there are a handful whom he especially needs to 'get my head round'. They are complex and potentially unstable. It will take an hour and a half to achieve that aim, and in the remaining two and half hours the spectrum of acuity and severity that he meets will be wide. Some of the patients will be medically fit, just waiting for a package of care. He tends, not unreasonably, to see them at the end of the round. But he *will* see them. They are his patients.

At twenty to one he looks down the list. There are still four patients to see. He has a regular meeting at one o'clock. He was late for it last time, and does not want to be late again. He asks for a précis of the patients' problems, and they are pretty much stable. One was admitted overnight, but the word is that they failed an occupational therapy assessment at the front door, and if not for that they would have been discharged immediately. 'Could you take a quick look?' he asks his registrar, Emma. 'Let me know if there are any real issues…medical issues.' He leaves the team. In truth, he left them half an hour ago. His attention began to slip, he began to ask the same question twice. The intellectual meat of the morning had been chewed and digested hours ago. He was now using reserves of enthusiasm that only professionalism drove him to access. But the team has done well. The week should proceed safely enough, now that they have the measure of their charges.

Emma and the rest of the team need to eat. She will see the new patient later, as promised. Did she promise? Well, she was asked and did not say no. That's the way it works. She has a clinic though, and it does not go as smoothly as she had hoped it would. At 4.50PM she bleeps the FY1, Luke, and asks him to make sure the new patient has been reviewed. He speaks his mind, does Luke, and he is just coming to terms with the requirements of the job – that is the ability to accommodate last minute requests and fit them into the sequence of the day. His job feels truly Sisyphean. Just as he is beginning to feel that he is getting on top of his list of tasks, another is added. 'I thought you…' he stops himself. 'OK, but if there's a problem, what should I hand over, the lumbar puncture or the new patient.' Emma replies quickly, 'Neither. But make sure the LP is done, please, that's crucial.'

Luke circles the name of the new patient at the bottom of his list. But he concentrates on the LP. He's done several, but cannot undertake them unsupervised. Emma would have looked on, but she remains tied up in clinic. His second option, Lucy, an experienced SHO on another firm, offered her time after lunch, but she is probably getting ready to go by now. He sees her, and sighs in relief when she makes the offer again. By 6.30PM they have done it. The samples are on their way. His day is almost over. Except for the new patient review.

A review. Just a review. But a *new* patient. That's the catch. To do it properly requires a 'from scratch' assessment of the presenting complaint and past medical history, and a physical examination. It's a 30 minute job, at least. He wants to do it. No, he wants to *have done* it. But now, at a quarter to seven, the task's magnitude has become inflated. What if it's complicated? What if the drug chart needs re-writing? It is unlikely. No-one has bleeped him about her during the afternoon. They must be truly stable – off legs at worst. Isn't that what they said on the ward round? – failed OT assessment, no 'medical' issues. Dr Blackburn wasn't interested. Luke recalled his far-away gaze, the evident lack of enthusiasm, 'Let me know…' he said, 'if there are any *real* issues…' Even consultants, with all their knowledge and experience, cannot achieve 100% of their work. Luke decides to take it on trust. The chances of that patient coming to mischief are *minimal*. Luke is not going to cut himself up about this one lapse. He's done so much today.

At three in the morning the on-call FY1 is called to see the patient. She finds him confused and septic, with clear signs of pneumonia. She is surprised such basic diagnosis could have been missed, and puts the fact that his chest x-ray and his blood tests have not been scrutinised down to the circumstances – the decision to admit was made late in the evening, and they must have been arranged just before he went to the ward. But she would have thought the results of those investigations (which include grossly elevated inflammatory markers) would have been seen on the ward round that day. Strange, she was sure Dr Blackburn himself went round on Mondays.

Right to be wrong: being comfortable with uncertainty

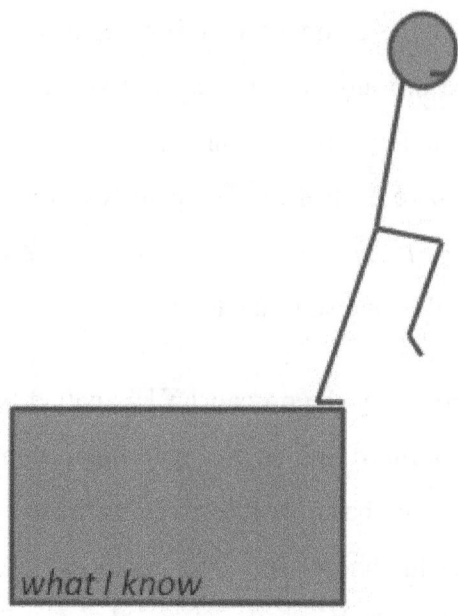

There are occasions when having the confidence to be wrong, and to be seen to be wrong, is advantageous to the patient.

Two cases:

I once saw a patient with signs of liver failure, but there was something about her that didn't make sense. No risk factors, no alcohol. She had too much fluid in the body ('overloaded'), and the veins in her neck were distended, a classic sign of heart failure. So, I thought, the liver signs could be secondary to the heart, and what she really needs is a cardiac assessment. I requested that assessment, and gave my reasons…but the cardiologist wasn't convinced it was her heart either. The story was all wrong, she had had a healthy heart scan within the last 6 months, and there were no risk factors! We talked, we went to and fro, and in order to ensure that an urgent echocardiogram was performed, I said,

'Well I'm pretty certain it's her heart, there is no history of liver disease, and at the moment heart failure is the most likely diagnosis…'

Thus I nailed my colours to the mast, and backed it up by writing unequivocally in the notes something along the lines of, '…*presentation most consistent with heart failure, needs urgent investigation…*' It was a form of brinkmanship, an unsubtle distribution of responsibility, such that my colleague felt compelled to attend urgently in order to check whether this patient's problem did indeed stem from heart failure.

The cardiologist attended an hour later, while I was still on the ward. He called me into the patient's bed space, behind the curtains, and showed me the images. The heart was beating perfectly normally. With equal emphasis, he wrote something along the lines of, '…valves and chambers normal, ejection fraction 60-65%, unchanged from __ /20__.' We discussed the details, and agreed that in fact what we were probably looking at was a case of fluid overload due to kidney failure. I went back to the notes, looked at my big, bold words on the page, and thought… *'You were completely, absolutely, wrong!'* But…but…by being bold, by taking a position, I achieved what was required - an urgent heart scan and a narrowing down of the differential diagnosis.

Another example. A patient with unexplained chest pain is admitted through the ED. It isn't a heart attack, it's not an ulcer, it's not a pulmonary embolism. The thought develops that it might be a thoracic aneurysm; potentially lethal, very hard to rule out. Do I really think it is? No, I'm not convinced, the pain is already settling, perhaps it *is* a bit of acid reflux, but I feel uncomfortable. She said it felt like a tearing sensation. She needs a scan. It's late. I'm going to have to make a good case to the radiologist.

'Hi, it's Dr_____. I've got a patient with chest pain, severe, and we've ruled most things out, but I'd like to exclude a dissecting thoracic aneurysm…no, the chest x-ray looks normal but I can't rely on that…the blood pressures in both arms are equal…'

I'm not doing well. How badly do I actually want this scan? If I'm not convinced (just concerned), so why push it? But if she *is* dissecting, and we miss it, she's as good as dead.

'…I just can't sit on her all night without ruling it out. We don't scan every chest pain, but the way she described it…it's the only remaining diagnosis I can think of.' The scan is agreed to. To back up my verbal conviction I write in the notes, '...plan: exclude dissection.' and I wait for the result. It is negative. Of course it is negative. Perhaps I used up a bit of credit with the radiologist, perhaps next time they won't take my request quite so seriously, but now, this evening, I achieved what I felt I needed to achieve.

Being wrong is nothing to be proud of, obviously. But what I describe here is a willingness to make a diagnosis and push hard for the investigations that are required to prove or disprove them. The process of forming a list of differential diagnoses and eliminating all but one (the actual diagnosis) will by its very nature involve barking up several wrong trees. Being wrong is therefore a necessary corollary to discovering the right answer. However, being wrong is not something that medical students or medical trainees are very comfortable with. Our training is focussed, entirely, on retrieving facts with accuracy and providing the 'right answer' immediately. Then, once we enter the real world, we encounter uncertainty, a whole series of possibilities stemming from each and every clinical encounter. It is physically impossible to pick out the right explanation for each collection of symptoms and signs. To make progress we must make a stab at the problem, have a go, test a series of theories, and, one by one, eliminate those that are wrong. If the discomfort that trainees feel in the face of uncertainty results in a form of paralysis, and the 'differential diagnosis' section at the end of the clerking is left blank, progress cannot be made. Progress requires an acceptance that medicine is uncertainty, a willingness to bark up those trees, and the maturity to absorb any sense of embarrassment that arises when the someone shouts down from the branches, 'Wrong one!'

Some free resources on uncertainty in medicine:

1) <u>Clinical uncertainty- Helping our learners</u> by Dale Guenter, Nancy Fowler and Linda Lee (Canadian Family Physician)

2) <u>Tolerance of Uncertainty and Fears of Making Mistakes Among Fifth-year Medical Students</u> by Maarit Nevalainen, Liisa Kuikka, Lena Sjöberg, Johan Eriksson and Kaisu Pitkälä (Family Medicine)

3) <u>The value of medical uncertainty?</u> By Caroline Welbery (Lancet) - On the role of art

4) <u>Uncertainty Is Hard for Doctors</u> by Danielle Offri (NEJM)

Patient complaints and the response arc

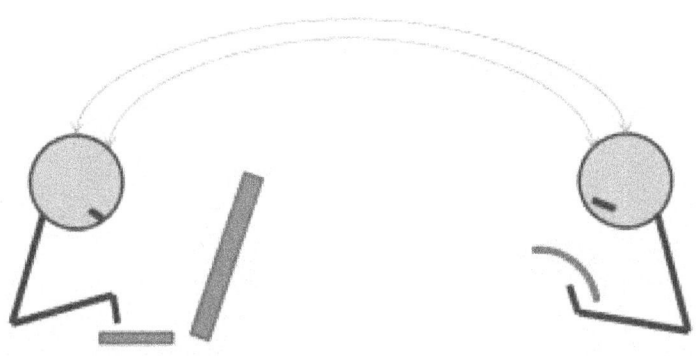

One of the painful duties that accompanies consultancy or general practice is that of responding to complaints. However good you are, or think you are, the huge numbers of patients that you see mean that complaints are inevitable. How doctors and nurses react to them is very important – both internally and externally. Their parent organisations must also respond, recognise patterns or extremes, and make changes where appropriate. But at the level of the individual, for all the important or ultimately constructive comments that these letters and emails contain, they are by their very nature critical. Criticisms will usually be directed at individuals, because care is delivered by individuals, and each must learn how to absorb the negativity and process the message such that something positive results. This is not easy, and I believe doctors or nurses who receive a complaint experience a dynamic reaction, the first phase of which involves anger and annoyance. This article describes one such arc, and interposes the thoughts of a fictional patient. The 68 year old lady, of extremely sound mind, was not informed that she was being discharged by her team, and was then left waiting for hours in a discharge lounge. Her consultant is required to respond.

oOo

Not another one

Yes, I remember the name. She didn't look happy when I walked past her on the day she left, something to do with not being informed, or transport delays, something. But we did a pretty good job, got her better

Come on!

> *"Is it worth writing this? I survived didn't I?*
> *But it was terrible, the way they left me…"*

Oh, that's trivial…it made no difference to her outcome…

The medicine was fine…this is nothing to do with me

204

I mean, I come into the office, open my emails, and what do I get – this! Just because my name was over the bed, it lands in my in-box.

"Nobody arranged transport. Nobody told me anything. They were desperate for the bed, I could tell..."

I can't be responsible for every little thing.

"But I'm going to. They need to know. A weaker patient, a frail little thing, could have caught their death of cold..."

Well, I'll write a response, but I'm not going to apologise.

"I can see him now, the consultant. He won't want to take any of the blame. But they were his nurses..."

I don't control staffing levels on the wards, I've got to focus on the hard stuff, the diagnosis, the treatment

"I'd say to him - don't you see, you represent the whole system? You were in charge of my care, and when I was ignored on the ward, when I was suddenly discharged and left waiting for transport for 4 hours in a drafty discharge lounge, I thought of you..."

Do I wake up in the morning and make a decision to deliver poor care? No! I do the best that I can in a pressurised NHS, an austere system…it's incredible that we do as well as we do. So I'm not going to take this to heart.

"But it's not about you, as such. It's about fixing your hospital."

OK…got to engage with this. Got to put down something constructive. It *was* a pretty rough experience by the sounds of it. I had no idea. Invisible to me, all that stuff, once I leave the ward.

"…and if it was your mother?"

Strange, really, I would have no idea this sort of thing happens if she hadn't written.

"Imagine then, how many don't write."

When's the last time I complained about anything? What does it take? A lot! This lady must have been incensed, to get home, to remember, to actually make the effort. Whenever I feel like complaining about anything it wears off after a couple of weeks. Can't be bothered.

...20 minutes later

Good. Done. Hardly a defence union issue! But I'll go have a word with the ward manager...let them know it spoilt what was otherwise a pretty efficient and successful patient journey...what's the point of me and my team getting all the medicine right if the patients feel abandoned when they've recovered? Makes the whole system looks bad.

> *"Well I'm pleased. It's almost as though we're talking!*
> *Such a shame we didn't talk at the time.*
> *None of this would have been necessary, I'm sure."*

Yes...I remember her better know, she was a lively lady. Perhaps I will apologise after all. Costs nothing

oOo

The key to accessing something positive, it seems to me, is the ability to exercise empathy over paper. One only needs to imagine how reluctant most of us are to complain about poor service in other walks of life. This is combined with a natural tendency to feel less angry with each passing day, when one has 'escaped' the situation that was so painful. If pen is put to paper, the intensity of dissatisfaction must indeed be considerable. And just as our role in any particular patient's poor experience is likely to represent a failure of the system rather than personal error, the letters that we receive are likely to be addressed to the system as a whole, rather than the individual named. The name may just be a representative symbol, and as such, perhaps we shouldn't allow the criticisms within to rile us too much. Less annoyance, more understanding - easy to say, not so easy to enact.

Hurricane Katrina and the DNR fallacy

It happened nearly a decade ago, and although the details were there to be read in articles and commentaries, the publication of Sheri Fink's book 'Five Days At Memorial' has provided an opportunity to explore the tragedy. However, for all the comprehensive detail, the author has been accused by the protagonist with the highest profile, Dr Anna Pou, of creating a fiction. She writes on her website,

> 'Now several years later Ms Fink has turned her article into a full length novel entitled "Five Days At Memorial [Hospital]" which concludes that scores of patients were euthanized by their doctors. The book is not only an insult to the self sacrificing doctors, nurses and other medical personnel who stayed in harm's way tending to patients in the most difficult of circumstances, but a disruption to the closure of this tragedy by suggestions to family members of patients who lost their lives that their loved ones were murdered.'

So what did happen? The narrative provided in Fink's earlier ProPublica article provides a clearer account than that presented in her perhaps over-detailed book, and I recommend it. However, this article is about the decisions that were taken well *before* the morphine and midazolam injections were given – namely the policy, hastily agreed in difficult circumstances, of equating DNR status with unsalvageable medical status.

First, a quick overview. Memorial Medical Centre (MMC) attracted attention soon after the waters receded because more people died there (45) than in any other New Orleans hospital. Suspicions grew that something unnatural had occurred. Indeed, one doctor had left during the flood unhappy about a perceived policy of euthanasia; *'I can't be part of anything like that.'* (p202) he said to a colleague.

After an investigation by the Medicaid Fraud Control Unit, evidence against Dr Pou was heard before a Grand Jury. It did not indict her on the one count of second-degree murder or the nine counts of 'conspiracy to commit second degree murder', and Dr Pou was released. The political atmosphere had become febrile by this time, and the accused doctor (two nurses who had also been accused were offered immunity for their testimony) received a great deal of popular support. Louisiana state's first term Attorney General, Charles Foti, failed to get re-elected because of his decision to pursue the charges.

The Triage

The hospital weathered the storm itself, but the floodwaters that rose following the failure of the levees isolated it entirely. Doctors and management team members met, and soon decided that the 'sickest, the ones most dependent on life support or mechanical aids, should go out first.' (p75) Normal clinical service could not be maintained and a senior physician decided that 'all but the most essential treatments and care should be discontinued.' (p81) Rationing of available resources (human and material) was therefore underway. Then (p92) Fink describes how, at the earlier meeting, 'doctors had established an exception to the protocol of prioritizing the sickest patients and those whose lives relied on machines. They had decided that all patients with Do Not Resuscitate orders would be prioritised last for evacuation.' Fink describes what DNR means, and emphasises that a 'DNR order meant one thing: a patient whose heartbeat or breathing stopped should not be revived', and a few lines later explains 'but the doctor who suggested at the meeting that DNR patient go last had a different understanding… [He] said he thought the law required patients with DNR orders to have a certified terminal or irreversible condition, and at memorial he believed they should go last because they had "least to lose" compared with other patients if calamity struck.'

As the evacuation process began, patients were triaged explicitly into 3 categories, '3's' being those judged to be 'very ill', or those with DNR orders. Pieces of paper with 1's, 2's and 3's were taped to patients' clothing, or written directly onto their gowns with thick black pens (p137). This link takes you to a disturbing picture in

Fink's ProPublica article; DNR is scrawled on an obtunded patient's gown, along with a '3'.

The DNR trap

This fallacy, that DNR = end of life, traps and confuses inexperienced nurses and clinicians in everyday clinical practise. Unless a DNR decision is made in the context of imminent death, I usually make a point of saying to the patient, and to ward staff, that 'this does not affect your treatment, we're still going to do our best to get you through this illness and home.' Care must be taken to prevent the impression that DNR means that we will relax, and not bother so much about the details. This danger is encapsulated in a slide taken from a recent presentation I gave on the subject.

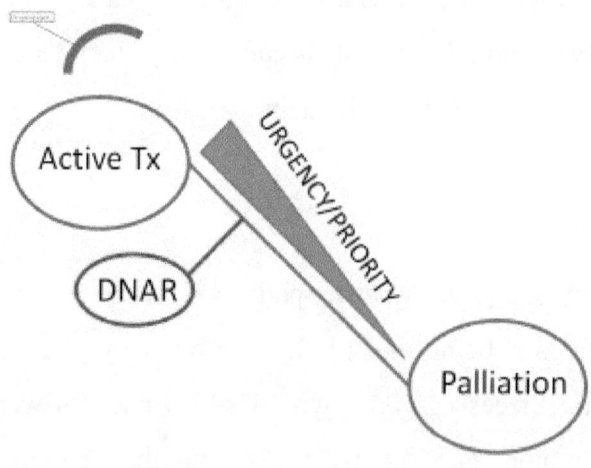

Despite this concern, in the absence of a disaster or a sudden need to ration personnel or equipment, it seems reasonable and achievable to promise that DNR will not affect other aspects of care. The question of limited resources will not come up. Or will it?

There is one scenario where <u>rationing may occur</u>, and that is at the cusp of admission to critical care units. Here, any signal that patients may be near the end of life, or not 'for everything', can influence the decision to transfer. It is not uncommon for ward doctors to delay DNR discussions for fear that the signal it gives to those who may be asked to review their patients and decide if organ support has a role. For not everyone can go to ICU. There are not enough beds. This is a form of rationing. Rationing of ICU beds exists, and has been well studied. Although rationing may not be the explicit reason for denying a patient admission, the perennial pressure on beds is very likely (in my view) to raise the bar of anticipated utility in the minds of those who must choose who passes through their unit's doors.

So perhaps Katrina does offer a lesson to those of us working in functioning health systems. DNR can be used as a label, and if care is not taken its meaning can be amplified into an awful shorthand (at handover for instance) such that it influences the general approach to care . For those of us advocating for more DNR decisions taken earlier after admission, in order to prevent resuscitation of highly frail an comorbid patients by default, the challenge remains – to balance pro-active decision making with protection against lazy thinking. This requires constant vigilance and energetic education.

oOo

Note: **Double effect**

The quintessential point in terms of the guilt, and one that can only be known by the people involved, is whether the primary intention of those involved in injecting patients was to kill or relieve distress. Some would contend that in certain, desperate circumstances, they are one and the same. A patient who is very near the end of life, and who is in pain or severely short of breath, will of course die sooner if morphine is administered. This is the well known double effect.

Note: **Reverse triage**

There are many reasons why some those triaged to leave last ultimately died. Moving bedbound, morbidly obese or ventilated patients to the helipad proved impossible, for instance. The concept of reverse triage, whereby the sickest go last, is commonly applied in the military setting, or in civilian catastrophes. It is not necessarily controversial. During the years since Katrina, new laws were passed in Louisiana indemnifying doctors against accusations of clinical neglect in the event of patients dying due to this policy.

Bed X

Earlier this month (June 2014) Dr Kate Granger closed the NHS Confederation annual conference with a powerful speech. In it she described being referred to by a nurse as 'Bed 7'. These two syllables seem to embody uncompassionate care. 'Bed' represents all that is awful about hospitalisation, apart from the illness itself. It represents horizontality, frailty, powerlessness and diminished autonomy. It brings to mind the issue of resource, the perennial pressure on beds, and the 'blockers' that cannot be housed in the community after they have recovered. And the number, '7', shows how people can become just one of many on the conveyor belt of sickness...a chore, a passing burden...in the minds of those who have forgotten what it is to act with compassion. Then, reflecting on this simple phrase, I realised something - I have may well have committed the same crime.

Can there be any excuse for referring to a patient by their bed number? The following, if not an excuse, may be an explanation.

When I started work in an A&E department I was immediately reminded of the days and evenings I had spent working as a waiter. The comparison seems trivial, but there are real similarities.

As a waiter I received a seemingly never-ending series of requests, backed up by the additional pressure of my customers' variously expressed frustration or annoyance. I had to decide who should be served first, or who should have their order taken next according to how urgent I thought their need was. Sometimes an unexpected piece of information would arrive which would lead me to prioritise one table above another even though they had taken their seats half an hour later (they had to get to a show, for instance). This might involve debasing myself before the (typically) knife-wielding chef, trying to convince him to let a table jump the queue. Sometimes a problem in the kitchen would force me to go and explain what had happened to the customers, while trying to avoid apportioning the blame to my colleagues. My mind would be teeming with parallel problems, but the hours would pass quickly and by 1 o'clock in the morning the room would be empty, the tablecloths thrown in laundry bins and the tips divided. Then, having eventually gone to sleep while the adrenaline was still subsiding, I might dream about tables, or tumbling forks, or I might see myself holding six plates, unable to move, glued to the carpet, while customers clamoured for food and shouted at me.

So, if we can accept that something as unimportant as a couple waiting for their steak can be compared to a sick patient waiting to be assessed in A&E, other similarities come to mind.

Just as table numbers dictated my movements in the restaurant, in A&E the code by which I organised myself, or was organised by the nurse in charge, related to cubicle numbers. Until I met a patient for the first time they would have no name. Their back story was unknown to me, they were no more than an item on a list, a set of notes in a tray. And until I met them for the first time their 'handle' was just a cubicle number. I would have read the initial triage assessment, I would be formulating an approach in my mind, but it would all be under the heading of simple, impersonal number.

Standing outside the curtain, as I responded to questions about other patients, I would signify my intention by saying, "Yes, but I'm just about to see cubicle 9." If this was overheard it might have sounded insensitive. Sometimes, I am sure, it *was* overheard. But surely no-one would expect a health care worker to use the term to a person's face!

It is conceivable that a health care worker might forget to dissociate the person they are just about to see from the label with which their mind has been 'handling' them. Perhaps, in an environment where the patient is new (such as A&E), such a slip, such thoughtlessness, might be forgiven. But for the patient on the ward who has already been in hospital for several days, and who has demonstrated that they are a whole person, and who is known to staff, such an error is less understandable. But for some staff the patient *will* be new. They may have just returned from a three day period off duty, and during handover the name, in the absence of the context of human contact, may not have displaced the easier label...the bed and bay number.

What *is* familiar to the nurse or doctor, through their many days on the ward, is the patient's location. In much the same way I knew the floor plan of my restaurant. My allocated sector for the night might include tables 9-18. I would immediately associate table 11 with that difficult approach around the foot of the stairs, or the tight squeeze by the potted palm, while laden with full glasses and plates. The bed number is not just a number, it is a location that the nurse has worked around for days and nights on end. It means something to the nurse, but it means nothing, of course, to the patient.

This (quite possibly flawed) analysis of human behaviour can only serve as an explanation, and is not an excuse for a lack of compassion. The thing that should stop the doctor or nurse translating a mere label into human communication is an understanding that the patient will be hurt by being referred to in such impersonal terms. This requires just a moment's reflection, reflection that should become habitual for someone working in health care, but a moment that might, possibly, be squeezed out by the pressure of work. Or by laziness. Or by dehumanisation. But it only takes a moment.

(And by the way, if the unfamiliar nurse were to say 'Hello, my name is...', the trap would immediately be avoided.)

Interactive Ward Ethics 3: Obedient

Having survived the challenges presented to her in <u>Collusion</u> and <u>Dangerous</u>, Nina must now negotiate her way through another nightmare week, in <u>Obedient</u>. Here she finds herself questioning a consultant's decision to set limits of care on a young patient with a life threatening problem. What should she do – obey, question, or seek alternative opinions? Each choice has its risks....and who is to say that she is right and her consultant is wrong?

As usual, you make the choices in this interactive blog. You can move backwards with the back arrow to escape from any cul-de-sacs. In the <u>Summing Up</u>, I explore the various issues faced by trainees in the still somewhat (necessarily?) hierarchical world of hospital medicine.

oOo

1.

Nina presented her patient to the consultant of the day. It was a Saturday evening. Her patient, Adrian, had alcoholic liver failure and looked awful. She described the history, the examination findings, the blood results. Dr Murphy shook his head and raised his eyes skyward.

The patient was 48 years old, and this was his first admission to hospital. He was bright yellow, his abdomen was full of excess fluid, and the tests showed that his kidneys were suffering also. Nina asked what should be done if he deteriorated.

"There isn't much that can be done, is there?" Dr Murphy replied, "I mean, he isn't getting a new liver is he? Only stopped drinking three days ago."

"But this is his first time in hospital. I've seen patients get admitted to intensive care for this…"

"He wouldn't benefit from that. He's too severe. In my experience, they do very badly indeed. We don't want to subject him to a long drawn out death on machines, do we? You've given him all the correct emergency treatment…see how he responds, but if he doesn't, better call the family in. If I'm still around I'll talk to them myself. They need to be put in the picture."

Nina wrote in the notes and paraphrased Dr Murphy's words. But she wasn't happy. She had seen patients like this get better.

A day later, on another night shift at 3AM, she was called to see Adrian. He was almost comatose. He was no longer passing urine. The jaundice was worse. She read her own handwriting in the notes – 'Ward based care, not for escalation to intensive care. Discuss resuscitation with family.' But still she wasn't happy. She picked up the phone.

Phone Dr Murphy at home (he is not on-call), go to 2

Phone the consultant on-call, go to 3

Refer to intensive care, go to 4

Commence end of life management, go to 5

2.

"Hello."

"Dr Murphy, it's Nina Charan, I'm sorry to phone you when you're not on-call."

"It's three in the morning!"

"I'm really sorry, I'd never normally do this."

"What's the emergency. Isn't Dr Lewis on call?"

"It's that man with alcoholic liver disease, he's got worse…"

"As I predicted."

"But…I wanted to double-check…are you sure we shouldn't send him to ICU?"

"Unless you know something about I don't, then yes, I'm sure!"

"OK."

"You don't sound OK. you obviously disagree."

"I just thought…"

"Look. I'm not there. You are. But my overall impression remains unchanged. That's all I can say. I'm not going to review him over the phone. The reason I made a decision, when we saw him together, was to make it easier for the on-call team to decide what to do when something like this happened. Goodnight!"

Refer to intensive care registrar anyway, go to 6

Leave it…give instructions for end of life care, go to 7

3.

"Dr Lewis, it's Nina the registrar on call. Sorry to call you, it's about a patient you won't have seen."

"Oh. What's the problem?" Nina told her. "Look, Nina, I don't know the patient, Dr Murphy gave a very clear opinion and he is extremely experienced. I think you should go with his decision."

"But…"

"You disagree. I realise that. I can't override his decision as I haven't seen the patient. Do I think young patients with alcoholic liver disease should be given a chance? Yes, sometimes. But there was clearly something about this patient that Dr Murphy felt meant that ICU wasn't appropriate. You could have challenged him at the time if you had reservations. Did you?"

"A bit. Not really."

"Well, it's too late for that now. So what are you going to do?"

"Nothing, I guess. I don't know."

Accept that there is nothing more to be done, go to 7

Find out more about the patient's background from relatives, go to 8

4.

The registrar came quickly, examined the patient, then emerged from behind the curtains. "There's lots we could do...but it says in the notes he's not for escalation. What's changed?"

"I think it's a bit premature to write him off. That's why I called you."

"But his consultant said he shouldn't."

"There's lots of evidence suggesting he could respond."

"But...what can I do? A decision has been made. And my consultant is going to say the same."

Speak to ICU consultant yourself, go to 9

Phone on-call medical consultant at home, go to 11

5.

Things were so much easier when the consultant had left such a clear directive. Despite the unarticulated murmurings of discontent in the back of her mind, Nina followed the instructions that had been given.

In the final analysis, it was not for her to question the opinion of a senior physician with far greater experience. She left the ward, having told the nurses that further calls were not to be made should Adrian's blood pressure drop.

Go to 10

6.

The intensive care registrar came quickly, examined the patient, then emerged from behind the curtains. "There's lots we could do...but he's not for escalation, it says so in the notes. What's changed?"

"I think it's a bit premature to write him off. That's why I called you."

"But his consultant said he shouldn't. And you've spoken to him...did he change his mind or something?"

"No, not really, but there's lots of evidence suggesting he could respond. I don't like to say it, but Dr Murphy is not a gastroenterologist...I was listening to a lecture on this situation the other day, it's recommended that these patients get full support until reversible factors like sepsis have been reversed..."

"But…what can I do? A decision has been made. And my consultant is going to say the same. Your consultant is still of the same opinion. Nothing has changed! Except he's a lot sicker."

Contact intensive care consultant, go to 13

Call on-call medical consultant, go to 14

7.

She said the words, she commiserated. Then Nina wrote something in the notes. It didn't reflect her opinion. But she suppressed her opinion. It was a junior opinion, an inexperienced opinion. The opinion of an optimist. She had expressed her reservation…subtly, without becoming strident or 'difficult'. She did not find confrontation easy to handle, and as she left the ward for the last time (she had given instructions that further emergency calls concerning Adrian were not to be made) it did occur to her that timidity, on her part, might have played a role in this patient's progress.

Go to 10.

8.

"Is the family coming in?" asked Nina of the ward nurse.

"On their way. The wife. Ex."

As Nina wrote up her notes the door to the ward opened and a woman entered. Nina knew that it must be Adrian's wife. Nina introduced herself and invited her into the relatives' room. They sat with the nurse. The wife, Lisa, started the conversation. She was agitated.

"No-one has spoken to me! No-one. You know nothing about him, nothing. And now he's dying!"

"I'm sorry about that. I don't think there has been an opportunity. But now we have time…what can you tell us about him?"

"That he wants to survive. He has done everything possible to stop drinking. He didn't drink for a year, and then last month, we split up…we had been talking about it for years…and he started again. But before that he was good, really good. His doctor said his liver had recovered. And he can recover again."

"Has he ever gone yellow before?"

"Never. His GP said there was liver damage but never said it would stop working completely."

Nina built up a full picture in her mind of Adrian's personal and medical history. It reinforced her impression that Adrian should have life supporting treatment if he needed it. She made up her mind…

Promise to get Adrian transferred to ITU, go to 15

Explain the differences of opinion among medical staff, go to 16

9.

The intensive care consultant was still in the building. He stayed over when on call. But he was asleep, and Nina nervously knocked on the door of the makeshift bedroom that had been set up in the department. He groaned and opened the door, rubbing his face and eyes.

"What's happening?"

"I want to get a patient with alcoholic liver disease into ITU but no-one agrees with me."

"How old is he?"

"48."

"That all. Do we know him?"

"No, first presentation."

"Drinking?"

"Yes."

"Bilirubin?"

"350."

"Kidneys?"

"No urine."

"Blood pressure?"

"85 systolic."

"Does he want to live?"

"This is the first time he's ever been sick."

"And who is saying no?"

"Dr Murphy."

"Ah…right. OK, tell the nurse in charge to prepare a bed."

Go to 12

10.

His blood pressure fell, his hands grew cold. His ex-wife sat by him, holding those pale fingers. Nina walked past several times, and had to stop herself averting her gaze. She found it difficult to make eye contact with the wife…because she knew, of she *felt*, that more could be done. But then again, Adrian was deteriorating quickly, which suggested that organ support on ITU may not have helped him. She presumed he had an overwhelming infection. He was receiving antibiotics…and that was the limit. Nina moved on again, to concentrate on the patients whom she could help.

Go to 22

11.

"Dr Lewis, it's Nina the registrar on call. Sorry to call you, it's about a patient you won't have seen."

"Oh. What's the problem?" Nina told her. "Look, Nina, I don't know the patient, Dr Murphy gave a very clear opinion and he is extremely experienced. I think you should go with his decision."

"But…"

"You disagree. I realise that. I can't override his decision as I haven't seen the patient. Do I think young patients with alcoholic liver disease should be given a chance? Yes, sometimes. But there was clearly something about this patient that Dr Murphy felt meant that ICU wasn't appropriate. You could have challenged him at the time if you had reservations. Did you?"

"A bit. Not really."

"Well, it's too late for that now. So what are you going to do?"

"Nothing, I guess. Though I'd better speak to the family…"

Tell the family that there is nothing more to be done, go to 7

Ask family more about the patient's background, go to 8

12.

With fluids and a small dose of vasopressor, Adrian's blood pressure improved and his kidneys began to function, producing measurable quantities of urine. The following morning she checked in on him again, before going home. As she left the unit Dr Murphy walked in.

"Dr Charan." he said, in a neutral tone.

"Dr Murphy. Sorry about last night."

"No, don't be, don't be. You must do what you think is in the patients best interest. But I *have* seen many patients like this one, and I do trust my own feelings on who will do well and who won't. We shall see. Let's hope for the best!"

As Nina walked away, she dwelt on her true opinion – that he knew nothing, was out of date, and was guilty of overlaying his own moral judgment on the decision he had made about Adrian's treatment. She would never dare say as much.

Go to 20

13.

The phone rang for minutes before it was picked up.

"Yes. What is it?"

Nina did not hesitate. She was in deep now, and was risking her reputation.

"I want to get a patient with alcoholic liver disease into ITU but no-one agrees with me."

"How old is he?"

"48."

"That all. Do we know him?"

"No, first presentation."

"Drinking?"

"Yes."

"Bilirubin?"

"350."

"Kidneys?"

"No urine."

"Blood pressure?"

"85 systolic."

"Does he want to live?"

"This is the first time he's ever been sick."

"And who is saying no?"

"Dr Murphy."

"Ah…right. OK, tell the nurse in charge to prepare a bed."

Go to 12

14.

"Dr Lewis, sorry…I need your help. I know you haven't seen him, but ITU won't admit this patient, and I feel very strongly that he should go. His family are equally sure he would want a trial of intensive care support…"

"It's not really up to them, is it?"

"But I think we have misjudged his medical situation, he's not end-stage, he's acutely unwell and there is reasonable chance he'll get better."

"So Dr Murphy was wrong, is what you are saying?"

"I am."

"Alright Nina, I'll call the ITU consultant."

She did, and three-quarters of an hour later Adrian was transferred.

Go to 12

15.

"I will make sure he gets the treatment he needs. I promise. I agree with you, he can get better again. His drinking is a reaction to the stress he has gone through recently."

Adrian's wife began to cry, and she thanked Nina.

— — —

Nina caught up with the ITU registrar. He was shaking his head.

"What?" asked Nina.

"You've committed us now."

"I know."

"Well I still can't guarantee anything." They both entered ITU. A phone rang, the sister answered it, and quickly passed the message to the registrar.

"There's a ruptured aneurysm in A&E. He's going to theatre now. We'll only have one bed after he has arrived."

The registrar shook his head again,

"My consultant won't want your chap in the last bed, I can guarantee it. You shouldn't have promised anything."

He rang the consultant and reported back to Nina,

"As I predicted…no way. Are you going to tell his wife."

Nina gave up. She had pushed against too many closed doors.

Go to 17

16.

Nina sighed, and decided to be frank.

"There's no easy way to explain this. We don't know what the best thing to do is."

"What do you mean?"

"I mean, there are always that *can* be done when patients develop such severe liver problems, but sometimes, if it is clear that things are going downhill very quickly, we come to the conclusion that it's not fair, on the patient, to put them through everything."

"Because they will die anyway you mean?"

"Yes."

"And you think Adrian is like that? Really?"

"It's not…it's not clear."

"Then if you aren't sure, you must do everything, mustn't you?"

"That's what I mean, the consultant who saw him when he first came in felt his chances of survival were very low indeed. He didn't feel going on life support machines would change that."

"But others disagree? You disagree, don't you."

"I haven't seen so many patients like Adrian."

"But I can tell you are not sure. And if you aren't sure, then you must give him the benefit of the doubt. Mustn't you."

Nina felt herself being squeezed; by her own conviction, by Adrian's wife and by the opposing force of the senior opinions that she had sought. She felt acutely uncomfortable.

"I'll…I'll…go and make some more calls."

Adrian's wife looked steely in her determination not to give up, but as Nina left the room her face softened.

"Doctor…I know this is difficult. I know this has been coming for many years. But he is too young."

Nina rang the intensive care registrar and emphasised the need for transferring Adrian to a higher level of care. She added what she knew about his wife's feelings, and what she understood of Adrian's attitude to medical treatment. But the registrar knew enough already. He knew that the true decision makers had made a negative assessment, and he would not be budged.

Give up and explain to Adrian's wife that nothing more can be done, go to 19

Phone the on call medical consultant, again! Go to 18

17.

Nina walked back to the ward. Adrian's wife stood by his bed. She asked Nina when Adrian would be transferred. Nina stood near her, and was close to speechlessness. As the silence expanded a mutual understanding developed. Adrian was unconscious, his brain swimming in ammonia and other toxins that could not be cleared by his damaged liver. Nina found speech, at last.

"I'm sorry. We can't take him there..."

"But you said."

Nina gave an explanation, and it sounded rational to her own ears. It was easy for her to repeat the words of others. There was very little conviction. She wondered if, when all this was over, Adrian's wife would reflect on the inconsistent messages that she had been given, and ask questions.

Go to Summing Up

18.

"Dr Lewis, sorry…"

"Again!"

"I need your help. ITU won't admit this patient, but I feel very strongly that he should go. His family are equally sure he would want a trial of intensive care support…"

"It's not really up to them, is it?"

"But I think we have misjudged his medical situation, he's not end-stage, he's acutely unwell and there is reasonable chance he'll get better."

"So Dr Murphy was wrong, is what you are saying?"

"I am."

"Alright Nina, I'll call the ITU consultant."

She did, and three-quarters of an hour later Adrian was transferred.

Go to 12

19.

"I'm sorry," said Nina, "It's too late."

"Is it? Really?" questioned Adrian's wife. What was her name again? Such was Nina's focus on the task in hand, to achieve Adrian's transfer, she had not given herself the space to be pleasant, or to make a human connection. Lisa…was that it?

"It is. I'm afraid he's dying."

"Yes, I can see it. I just hoped…that he would have the chance to fight it, for a bit longer…"

Go to 10

20.

Three days later Nina saw one of the gastroenterology consultants, Dr Redburn, leaving the intensive care unit. She noticed her and said,

"Sorry Nina, your patient's died. Massive bleed. Didn't have a chance, they tried to tamponade him but he went into DIC. Nothing to do I'm afraid."

Later in the day she met Dr Murphy. He had been informed. He was conciliatory, but she picked up a hint of condescension.

"Nina, I don't want to make a big thing out of this, but I do want you to learn from it. About why I made the decision not to escalate. There was something about him. Perhaps it was his nutritional status, perhaps there are unmeasurable signs that cannot be clearly described. It's called experience, and I have more of it than you."

So Nina reflected. But, by the end of the reflections, she decided that next time, in the same situation, she would act in the same way. Perhaps, later in her career, she would allow nihilism to influence her decision-making. But not yet.

Go to 21

21.

Nina walked the corridors nervously. She had put her head above the parapet, and she had gone with her conviction. But she had disobeyed an instruction, there was no escaping that fact. No new information had been given to her that influenced the medical decision, yet she had valued and responded to her own opinion above that of her consultant.

Three consultants sat drinking coffee. Dr Murphy, Dr Redburn the gastroenterologist, and Dr Canvey, Nina's supervisor.

"It's insubordination, in my opinion. She just ignored my instructions. What is the point of doing consultant ward round to making decisions if those decisions are ignored?" said Dr Murphy.

"As you admitted yesterday John," said Dr Canvey, "only she knew what the patient looked like in the moment. You can't second-guess her interpretation of the patient's condition. I accept you had made some overarching decisions, but it was a dynamic situation. You can't blame her."

"Well I do. The poor patient was subjected to half a week in intensive care, and look what happened to him. He died anyway. My impression was correct, he didn't have a chance."

"He did have a chance John," said the gastroenterologist, "statistically he had a reasonable chance. He was young, his liver dysfunction was acute…"

"He bled to death didn't he? He had varices, he must have had the condition for years."

"Yes, he had long-term liver damage, but the deterioration was acute and he might have responded to steroids if he'd survived long enough to have them prescribed. The bleed was unpredictable, and on another day, who knows, perhaps it could have been stopped."

"But I was right."

"Yes on this occasion, but next time, a patient of the same age with the same presentation might well survive. None of us can pretend to know what determines who survives. I think Nina made the right decision. If someone dies in intensive care it doesn't mean it was a waste of time. I back her up on this one."

Nina's supervisor now asked, "Are you saying you disagree with John's impression? You would have given different instructions of that ward round?"

"I think so. But it's my specialty, I'm trained to see opportunities to make patients better who have conditions that those with less experience tend to lump into one. John will identify patients with chest problems who can be salvaged who I would overlook. There is variability in the hospital, there are different areas of expertise, we can't get around that. But Nina, she's in training, and she is probably more in touch with current evidence that any of us. So give some credit. She made a decision, and she stuck to it. He didn't suffer that much. He didn't suffer at all."

Go to Summing Up

22.

Nina's bleep went off. She rang the number and recognised the voice of the hospital's new-ish gastroenterologist. She was known to be aggressive, medically – an enthusiastic advocate of maximum intervention for patients with liver disease. Nina had been expecting this call.

"Nina. It's Dr Redburn. I'm ringing about that patient from last night."

"Ah…yes."

"I know Dr Murphy set limits of care for him, and I wouldn't expect you to go against his decision, but you should know…"

"I do know."

"Why didn't you call me? I'd have spoken to ITU."

"It was the middle of the night."

"Sometimes you have to do uncomfortable things Nina. I'm not asking to be called every night, but for him…it might would have been understandable. These patients should be always be considered, at the very least, for ITU. Enough said."

Go to Summing Up

Summing Up – Obedient

Hospital medicine, despite the encouragement given to trainees to speak up and challenge, remains hierarchical. I don't think this reflects old-fashioned views among consultants, more a realisation that medicine is a genuine apprenticeship. The trainee is absorbing knowledge at all times, and working out how to turn what they observe into improved practise. It is a downhill transfer of skill and experience, and because of this discussing, let alone challenging, the decisions that they see does not come easily.

Obversely, established consultants must change over time in order to keep up to date. Often, the only way they will learn about the need to change will be by listening to their trainees. This view does not make picking up the phone at three in the morning any easier, but sometimes, in situations where lives are at risk, it will be justifiable in order to make it clear that things have moved on.

So what would I have done here, if I truly believed that Adrian had a reasonable chance of surviving on ITU? I would have been too nervous to ring Dr Murphy when he was not on-call. Hospitals should be able to run safely with the staff who are rota'd on, although there are rare occasions when specific knowledge has to be accessed and only one person has it. I would probably have argued my case with the intensive care team, and would have been explicit about why I thought the original decision was wrong. It does require a good understanding of the evidence, or of current guidelines, to be able to do this, and just 'having a feeling' that organ support should be offered is probably not enough. Of course it is essential to obtain the patient's view about treatment, but if they are cognitively impaired by their disease the best that can be achieved is a relative's 'substituted judgment'. This is not infallible as a guide, and, as Dr Lewis said over the phone in the scenario, the decision to go to ITU is not one that can be made by the family. It is a medical decision. If I got no joy from ITU I would have called Dr Lewis, the on-call consultant at home, and if she too felt that ward based care was appropriate, based in the information available, then perhaps I would have submitted to the greater experience the two consultants in combination. After all, one cannot go crusading around the hospital indefinitely.

But, what if I knew, if I was certain, that some factor, some piece of evidence or laboratory result suggested that barring Adrian's entry to ITU was tantamount to negligence? Then...I would have no choice...I would have had to make a terrible fuss, stamp my feet and wake everyone up! To do this requires utmost confidence in one's medical opinion, and trainees, being trainees, seldom have this.

www.ingramcontent.com/pod-product-compliance
Lightning Source LLC
Chambersburg PA
CBHW051212170526
45166CB00005B/1854